THE Women'sHealth® FITNESS FIX

QUICK HIIT WORKOUTS, EASY RECIPES, AND STRESS-FREE STRATEGIES FOR MANAGING A HEALTHY LIFE

JEN ATOR, CSCS
Fitness Director of Women'sHealth®

D1008912

© 2017 by Rodale Inc.

All rights reserved. No part of this publication may be reproduced or transmitted in any form or by any means, electronic or mechanical, including photocopying, recording, or any other information storage and retrieval system, without the written permission of the publisher.

Rodale books may be purchased for business or promotional use or for special sales. For information, please e-mail: BookMarketing@Rodale.com.

Women's Health is a registered trademark of Rodale Inc.

Printed in the United States of America
Rodale Inc. makes every effort to use acid-free ∞, recycled paper ♻.

Photographs by Beth Bischoff and Mitch Mandel/Rodale Images
Book design by Carol Angstadt

Library of Congress Cataloging-in-Publication Data is on file with the publisher.
ISBN 978-1-63565-016-7

Distributed to the trade by Macmillan
2 4 6 8 10 9 7 5 3 1 paperback

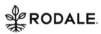

RODALE.

Follow us @RodaleBooks on

We inspire health, healing, happiness, and love in the world. Starting with you.

No success is ever just about a finish line—
it's about the people who are there for you
every step of the race, cheering you on,
picking you up, and making you feel like a
winner regardless of the final score.

———————————

To my amazing family and friends . . .
thank you for continuing to be there
to share in every accomplishment,
big and small.

Contents

PART III / KEEP IT GOING

Introduction

IN MY 8-PLUS YEARS AS THE FITNESS DIRECTOR AT *WOMEN'S HEALTH,* I've spoken to thousands (if not hundreds of thousands) of people about dieting and working out. The topic comes up in nearly every conversation I have. From hot new fitness trends or the latest diet craze to my own diet and exercise routine—you name it and I've been asked about it. And I'm constantly amazed by how many people still believe "the answer" is out there: the one workout that will finally flatten their belly, that one diet that will shed those last 10 pounds. They just haven't found it.

To these hopefuls, I say this: Healthy living really isn't as difficult, complicated, or time-consuming as it's always seemed. You'd never know it, thanks to the revolving door of new diet and fitness crazes (each claiming to hold the key to the best-kept secret), but there is no magic pill that will cure all of your fitness woes. It's not the latest popular DVD, hot new guru, or celeb-loved juice cleanse. What most people don't realize—or maybe can't accept—is it's not necessarily their workout program or diet that's broken: It's their mentality. We've largely become a society that views "being healthy" like it has an on-off switch. Even the most valid diet program or workout plan is just a band-aid, a temporary solution. Sure, it can get you results, but in most cases it's not designed to help you maintain those results forever. Why? Because it's not designed to change your lifestyle—or your outlook.

Entrepreneur and philanthropist Naveen Jain once said: "Don't follow the routines of people who are successful, follow their thought patterns," and that quote has always resonated with me. He was likely talking about business, but his words apply so perfectly to fitness and dieting. Lots of diets *can* work. Lots of fitness programs *can* work. That's not to say the methods don't matter—they absolutely do. Which is why inside these pages you'll find all the pieces you need for successful and lasting weight loss. These strategies are practiced by the country's leading fitness experts, tested by the world's top researchers, and proven by everyday women like you and me. But like Naveen said, it's more than just following a set of actions: To be truly successful, it's about looking at the "why" behind their approach, understanding the reasoning and the perspective behind the choices they make and the behaviors they practice.

In Part I, we'll focus on the things that need changing. We'll look at some of the top reasons diets fail, along with the "secrets" that successful dieters (aka people who manage to maintain their health, weight, and fitness levels year after year, decade after decade) have in common. I'll give you a hint right now: They're far more straightforward and manageable than you may believe.

In Part II, we'll drill down on the actionable steps you can take to become one of those forever-fit people. Unlike some diet and fitness books, you won't find one organized workout or meal plan to follow. Instead, you'll get a menu of efficient and effective ideas you can tweak and tailor to your schedule, your personal preferences, and your goals. Because this book is more than just getting you great results once: This book is about helping you establish a new mentality and flexible exercise and diet plans that will allow you to get great results—and keep them up forever.

Part III is all about how to keep it going. One of the biggest reasons diets fail is pretty obvious: They weren't built to last. There's no protocol for what to do after you finish those first perfectly planned-out days. This section is about thinking long term and managing different obstacles that come your way as you maintain a healthy, active lifestyle—from hectic schedules and injuries to workout motivation and goal setting.

This isn't a diet book.

It won't get you dramatic results in 30 days or less.

It isn't the magic pill.

But my hope is that it will help you see fitness and healthy eating through a different lens—one that actually feels manageable and maintainable.

DON'T LET YOUR PAST DICTATE YOUR FUTURE. IT'S NEVER TOO LATE TO BECOME BETTER.

PART I

MAKE
THE
CHANGE

1 / Before You Move a Muscle

LET'S GET SOMETHING STRAIGHT: I'm not here to challenge your time-crunched schedule—and I'm certainly not going to make you feel guilty for putting off a workout from time to time. Fitness is in my job title, and even I'm not immune to daily time-management (and motivation) struggles. I spend long hours behind a desk, I work late, and I hardly ever get a full 8 hours of sleep. I actually enjoy and look forward to working out, yet even I'm guilty of letting weeks pass without going to the gym. I get where you're coming from—because I'm right there with you.

Time (or lack of it) is an easy thing to blame, but the truth is that your schedule is not the biggest thing stopping you from feeling leaner, stronger, and more energized—it's your mentality. And that's what I'm hoping to change right out of the gate.

Too many women fall into an all-or-nothing mindset when it comes to diet and exercise. To them, these things are simply a means to an end. In an effort to see lightning-fast, jaw-dropping results, they seek out extremes: They spend hours at the gym, nix every "bad" food in the book, count every calorie. There's next to no room for error. In short, women demand perfection.

The problem? Almost anyone can suffer through a brutal month of over-training and calorie restriction and lose a few quick pounds, but research has continually proven that people can't keep it up for long periods of time. It's simply not sustainable—physically or mentally. In most cases, at some point—after a few days, weeks, or maybe months—this enthusiastic diligence slows (or worse, backfires), causing women to spiral back to the "nothing" end of the effort spectrum. Cue a single roadblock—like a week off from the gym or that pint of Ben & Jerry's you swore you wouldn't polish off—and all of a sudden the wheels come off. When women take an all-or-nothing approach, they see one slipup as complete failure and they give up.

While small fluctuations on the scale are normal, this start–stop pattern usually leads to a significant increase or decrease in body weight (generally 10 pounds or more), and it's usually not a one-time deal. Experts refer to this as weight cycling—you know it as yo-yo dieting.

According to a study published in the journal *American Psychologist,* dieters successfully lost up to 10 percent of their weight within the first 6 months on any number of diets; the problem is, nearly two-thirds of dieters put the weight back on (sometimes gaining even more) within 5 years.

As if the roller-coaster scale wasn't tough enough, weight cycling can actually change your physiology, increasing a hunger hormone called ghrelin and decreasing a fullness hormone called leptin. The result: You feel hungrier and less satiated, and over time, the more diets you've been on, the harder it becomes to lose the weight. Researchers from Columbia University in New York City found that dieting can actually slow your resting metabolism and make it harder to maintain a stable weight post-diet. They reported that dieters may burn up to one-quarter fewer calories during exercise than those naturally at the same weight.

Just as yo-yo dieting hurts your waistline, having an on-again, off-again relationship with working out wreaks havoc on your health: People who gained 14 pounds in a month by exercising less and eating more were still up nearly 7 pounds from their original weight 30 months later, despite going back to their healthier patterns, according to a study in *Nutrition & Metabolism.* An irregular exercise pattern can raise your body's natural set point (the weight your biological system naturally tries to maintain) and make it harder to dip below that number. And research shows that bouts of vigorous exercise followed by weeks of inactivity can increase fat levels and put excess strain on your cardiovascular system.

A "NEW" WAY OF THINKING

But your relationship with healthy eating and exercise doesn't have to be so hot and cold. In fact, ignoring strict guidelines could be the secret to a successful slim-down. A study published in the *International Journal of Obesity* found that people with a flexible approach to eating—one that allows for sweets and other perceived slipups—had a better track record of maintaining weight loss than dieters with an all-or-nothing strategy. And research shows that consistent exercisers who see working out as a part of their lifestyle, rather than a way to change their appearance, have the most success keeping weight off. So if some days you're too busy for even a few minutes of exercise or you slip up from your diet, you can give yourself a break. Because here's the bigger picture: It's what you do most of the time—not all of the time—that makes a difference. When overweight subjects in a study made several small lifestyle shifts—such as eating breakfast, having as many veggies as they'd like with each meal, and watching TV for only as long as they'd exercised that day—they dropped an average of 8 pounds in 2 weeks. And they kept it off.

The reason: When you focus on doing things that are fast, easy, effective, and, yes, even enjoyable, you're more likely to repeat them. It's the root of what experts call the Self-Determination Theory, which boils down to this: The more you do stuff you like to do (and not what you think you should do), the more you'll keep doing it. The benefits of this intrinsic, or internal, motivation have been proven in studies across the board—from education to health care to parenting. In exercise research, intrinsically motivated exercisers were more likely to continue working out for 6 months or more than those who were nagged by friends or family.

At the heart of true long-term success is repetition. When you take a look at the principal achievement among people who seem to always be in phenomenal shape, you'll likely see a common denominator: They have made being active and eating healthy a consistent part of their way of life. It isn't a switch they turn on before beach season or a big event and then shut off as soon as it's over. By following their lead, eventually what you eat and how much you move will become nearly unconscious habits, rather than constant daily stressors. Instead of throwing off your routine, you will find that these healthy decisions have become an integral part of it.

That's not to say that it ever gets easier to find time: Researchers at the University of Alberta in Edmonton found that even for people who love to exercise, scheduling regular workouts can still be a challenge. A few years ago, I was out to dinner in New York City with the incredibly fit, active, and vibrant LaJean Lawson, PhD, a 63-year-old exercise scientist. I asked her, "What's your secret to staying in such great shape?" Her answer was simple: Identify your "basic threshold" of fitness that is impossible to fail. Early on, Lawson decided she had to claim an unrelenting identity as a fit person, and she needed to perform an intentional fitness activity daily. Her basic threshold: one pullup or two full pushups. So at the end of every day, whether she is sick, or traveling, or crazy with work deadlines, she still does one of those two things. It may not sound like much, but, in less than 15 seconds a day, it has enabled her to maintain a very long streak of being a continuously active person.

While I loved the philosophy and her inspiring attitude, I was skeptical; there was no way something so basic could work for me. "She probably is just super petite naturally or has an unnaturally speedy metabolism," I thought. I might have doubted her theory, but I gave it a shot anyway. My first basic threshold: walking to and from work (about 25 minutes each way), rather than taking a cab or the subway. It didn't take long to notice that instead of feeling defeated for missing a spin class, I was proud that I kicked off my heels and hiked home—even if it was raining, snowing, or late. Was the effort comparable? Of course not, but it helped shift my mindset and it made me feel like I was still on track.

Lawson's modest approach stuck with me, and I have repeatedly tested—and proved—its effectiveness. (Walking is now part of my normal daily routine.) Every few months I shake up that bare minimum: Sometimes I choose one simple exercise and do 10 or 15 reps before I hop in the shower in the morning; other times, I simply commit to spending a few minutes foam rolling before bed. These activities don't outweigh or replace my workouts, but they help connect the dots in between missed sessions and breed confidence rather than frustration. As Lawson so perfectly told me, "In the end, being able to claim your identity as a 'fit person' is as much a state of being as it is a state of doing."

This is so incredibly important: For people who successfully maintain active and healthy lives for years and decades, their daily behaviors don't change how they see themselves; they don't impact their self-worth. They're still active, healthy people. Even if they haven't been to the gym in weeks. Even if, in one indulgent day, they ate cake for breakfast and pizza for dinner. They don't beat themselves up or give up on their goals and healthy habits because they made one mistake or temporarily lost sight of their goals. It doesn't change how they think of themselves as people.

While you may be skeptical, I can promise that this is the biggest shift you can make for lasting results. You have to stop thinking, "Once I lose this weight, I'll be happy" or "Once I can fit into this size dress, I'll feel good about myself." That all-or-nothing, backward way of thinking is keeping you in this on-and-off cycle. Fake it till you make it if you have to, but stop being so damn tough on yourself and start seeing the good. Start seeing what you do right and well, and start appreciating your body for its strength, power, and potential—because it really does matter. Case in point: In a study at the Technical University of Lisbon in Portugal, women who were counseled to improve their body image lost a higher percentage of weight than those who weren't. Poor body image can lead to emotional eating and anxiety, which sabotage weight loss. In fact, researchers at the Miriam Hospital Weight Control and Diabetes Research Center in Providence, Rhode Island, found that internal emotional triggers—such as depression or stress—pose a larger obstacle to weight loss than external ones—for example, eating more because dinner is served buffet-style.

There are always going to be external obstacles we can't predict or control. That's just a given; that's life. Whether something transforms into anxiety has to do with your perception of the situation. Two different people can be met with the same challenge—say, that buffet-style dinner—but their reactions and impulses may be completely different based on their personalities or their mindsets. One person might feel overwhelmed, or even stressed, by all the choices—and quickly abandon her usual healthy eating habits because, "Oh well, the damage is done"—while the other may calmly take a lap around the buffet to see what's available before deciding what sounds good, then slowly enjoying every bite, just like she would at any other meal. Make that your top priority: Controlling the things you can, which, more often than not, will mean controlling the internal triggers that inevitably pop up. That's something you can do every single day. And if you want to score a better body, a happier mind, and a healthier relationship with diet and exercise—it's something you *need* to do every single day.

FIND YOUR STARTING LINE

I know what some of you might be thinking: If people aren't willing to dedicate an hour a day to their health and fitness goals, then they don't truly value them. A few of you may even be thinking that people looking for shortcuts don't deserve the same level of results as those who put in more work. These are fair points. I agree that people will find time to prioritize the things that are most important to them.

But people also make time for the things they enjoy the most. And I think that many people who allot an hour or more per day to, let's say, working out, are people who genuinely enjoy doing it. It goes beyond the fact that they value their health and their body—that time they find to work out is something they look forward to because it's an activity they truly like.

I'm in no way saying that long workouts and super-clean diets are bad or ineffective—I'm just saying that you don't have to do them to get in great shape. The word to remember for lasting results is *consistency*. (To get better, it's *progress*.) Especially for beginners or those who seem to always fall off the wagon, the initial focus should be on learning simple exercise and nutrition tools and being consistent with them. To do this, starting with 10 minutes of exercise a day is a better idea than jumping straight into longer or tougher workouts. Over time, you may even learn to love it.

Look at this book as a starting place. The goal is to build lasting habits—not burn out. Once you've done that, by all means, progress! Challenge yourself to longer, tougher workouts. Hone your lean-eating patterns a little bit more. If at any time you fall off the wagon or hit a setback, come back to this book as a way of resetting and getting back on track.

QUICK TIPS:
STRESS

1 **Feeling anxious? Work out, don't veg out.** A study in *Medicine & Science in Sports & Exercise* found that not only did people score lower on anxiety tests right after working out, but they also kept their cool 30 minutes later. Physical activity boosts blood flow to the parts of the brain that keep you calm, say study authors. But consistency is key: A single bout of sprinting on the day of a high-stress event could cause more strain than relief if your body isn't used to that level of intensity.

2 **Take a quick lap before a stressful event.** Ten minutes of exercise is all it takes to reduce anxiety before a nerve-wracking social gathering or work meeting. In a study, a 10-minute walk or jog helped people see their environments as less threatening.

3 **Work out after work.** Exercising for 15 minutes after a stressful workday may help you eat 125 fewer calories than if you were to veg out.

Study authors think the sweat session could distract you and nudge you to make healthier choices.

4 **De-stress your work environment.** People who clocked more than 40 hours a week or who feel threatened, bullied, or harassed at work are more likely to be obese than other employees, reports the *American Journal of Preventive Medicine.* This may be true in part because stress from a hostile environment can make you crave junk food and trigger hormones that increase fat deposits—not to mention that marathon workdays could shrink your gym time, say study authors.

5 **Avoid sympathetic stress.** Twenty-four percent of people experienced a significant jump in cortisol levels—the fight-or-flight hormone—after watching videos of others in tense situations. Elevated cortisol levels over time can put individuals at higher risk for diabetes,

QUICK TIPS:
STRESS *(cont.)*

weight gain, gastrointestinal issues, immune system suppression, cardiovascular disease, fertility problems, and other issues.

6 Stop eating your feelings. Yeah, it's real. A new study shows why we might not be able to stop eating when we're down in the dumps. German researchers found that after mildly depressed people watched movie clips with emotionally charged scenes, they were more sensitive to sweet, bitter, and sour tastes but far less able to discern fat, compared to when they watched neutral videos.

7 Develop good habits. When you're overwhelmed, you're likely to fall back on habits—including good ones. In a *Journal of Personality and Social Psychology* study, people who regularly ate unhealthy foods went for more junk when under the gun, but A+ eaters kept up their healthy eating patterns, even during frenzied times. Stress tires the brain, so we do what takes the least mental effort, say study authors.

8 Meditate to moderation. People who meditated for as little as 8 minutes per day were better able to control their desire to pig out and less likely to give in to emotional eating triggers, according to research from Rush University Medical Center. The practice helps people learn to be comfortable with, say, boredom or anxiety, rather than trying to get rid of the feelings with food.

THE BEST THING YOU CAN DO IS GET OUT OF YOUR OWN WAY.

2 / Taking the First Step

ONE OF THE MOST underappreciated fitness fads lately? All-day movement. No, seriously. You see, while the advancements we've made in the tech world are nothing short of inspiring, and certainly helpful, they're not necessarily improving every aspect of our lives. Mayo Clinic researchers estimate that we burn 1,500 to 2,400 fewer calories per day (per day!) than we did just 50 years ago.

Seems crazy, right? Consider this stat: According to a poll of nearly 6,300 people by the Institute for Medicine and Public Health at Vanderbilt University in Nashville, Tennessee, it's likely that you spend a stunning 56 hours a week sitting—staring at a computer screen, working the steering wheel, or collapsed in a heap in front of your high-def TV. And it turns out women may be more sedentary than men, since they tend to play fewer sports and hold less active jobs.

This downtime is now so prevalent that it has paved the road for a new area of medical study called inactivity physiology, which explores the effects of our increasingly butt-bound lives, as well as a deadly epidemic researchers have dubbed "sitting disease."

When muscles—especially the ones in your lower body—are immobile, circulation slows and you burn fewer calories. Key flab-burning enzymes responsible for breaking down triglycerides (a type of fat) simply start switching off. Sit for a full day and those fat burners plummet by 50 percent. The less you move, the less blood sugar your body uses; research shows that for every 2 hours spent on your backside per day, your chance of contracting diabetes goes up by 7 percent. Your risk for heart disease goes up, too, because enzymes that keep blood fats in check are inactive. Inactivity can also raise hell on your posture and spine health: Your hip flexors and hamstrings shorten and tighten, while the muscles that support your spine become weak and stiff. Not to mention that, with less blood flow, fewer feel-good hormones are circulating to your brain, making you more prone to depression.

More bad news: Even if you exercise, you're not immune to these effects. We've become so sedentary that 30 minutes a day at the gym may not do enough to counteract the detrimental effects of 8, 9, or 10 hours of sitting. This is one big reason why so many women still struggle with weight, blood sugar, and cholesterol woes despite having consistent workout routines.

A LITTLE GOES A LONG WAY

One of the most important and life-altering discoveries to come out of recent exercise research is that getting into shape isn't an all-or-nothing proposition. In fact, you can make a significant impact on your waistline without ever stepping foot in the gym.

How's that possible? Well, slaving away inside your body—right this minute—is your very own personal trainer working tirelessly to help you burn calories and shed fat. It's called your metabolism, and it's the sum of everything your body does. Each time you eat, enzymes in your body's cells break down the food and turn it into energy that keeps your heart beating, your mind thinking, and your legs moving during a grueling workout. The faster your metabolism runs, the more calories you burn. The more you burn, the easier it is to drop pounds. But while many people blame a sluggish system for their weight-loss woes, here's a secret: You can make your metabolism work harder—a lot harder—24 hours a day.

You see, to some degree, our bodies hum along at a preset speed determined by gender and genetics, but there's still plenty of wiggle room. You have a huge amount of control over your metabolic rate. You can't affect how many calories it takes to keep your heart beating, but science shows that you can burn an extra 500 to 600 calories a day by exercising properly and eating right.

Mayo Clinic researchers have extensively studied the impact of activities like folding laundry, tapping your toes, standing up, even having sex—what they refer to as daily nonexercise activity thermogenesis (NEAT), or the energy you burn doing everything but exercise. They found that lean participants moved an average of 150 minutes more per day than overweight participants did—enough to burn 350 calories. A University of Missouri study found that staying on your feet blasts up to 60 calories more per hour than sitting. Adding these simple activities can help stave off the 1- to 2-pound weight gain most women experience every year—and it can keep your metabolism buzzing the way nature intended it to. In fact, research has found that regardless of how much moderate to vigorous exercise a person does, those who take more breaks from sitting throughout the day have slimmer waists (by more than 2 inches!), lower BMIs (body mass indexes), and healthier fat and sugar levels in their blood than those who sit the most. Not to mention that getting off your butt for roughly an additional hour a day can decrease stress and heighten your mood, energy, focus, and productivity, according to the Centers for Disease Control and Prevention. Oh, and this: A woman can add an average of $5\frac{1}{2}$ years to her life expectancy—just by being active in her free time.

Commit this phrase to memory: Any amount of exercise is better than none, and research consistently proves that more frequent bursts of intense physical activity can produce the same muscle-building, fat-blasting, health-boosting benefits as the long-recommended 30 minutes a day. Studies have found that brief, vigorous workouts improve your body's ability to control blood sugar and lower blood pressure more than longer, less frequent sweat sessions; researchers in Denmark found that participants who completed shorter workouts burned more calories than those who logged more drawn-out ones.

What's more, the results seem to be cumulative, meaning you may get more points for repeated efforts—a set of squats in the morning, a brisk walk at lunch, and some pushups before bed—than for a single marathon cardio session at the gym. And because a person can go all out for 60 seconds but not 60 minutes, mini workouts can actually be more effective at sending your metabolism into overdrive, increasing your calorie burn during and after each fitness blast. Still not convinced? Here are seven ways short sweat sessions can improve your life.

INCREASE STRENGTH

Just three 15-minute weight workouts a week can double a beginner's strength, report scientists at the University of Kansas. Not to mention that, unlike the average person who quits a new program within a month, 96 percent of the study participants easily fit the short workouts into their lives.

DECREASE PERCEIVED EFFORT

If you think your workout is too hard, you're less likely to lose weight, reports the journal *Obesity*. When women were asked to rate how much a treadmill workout kicked their butts, those who ranked it the toughest packed on the most pounds a year later. The study's authors found that when you have a negative experience with exercise, you're less apt to do it.

BLAST BELLY FAT

In an Australian study, women who cranked out high-intensity interval training 3 days a week for 20 minutes (for 15 weeks) shed more fat than those who exercised for 40 minutes at a lower intensity over the same period.

IMPROVE EFFICIENCY

Previously inactive women who exercised four times a week gained just as much fitness in 16 weeks as those who did six workouts a week. What's more, they actually burned more total calories each day, reports a study in the journal *Medicine & Science in Sports & Exercise*. What gives? Those who exercised more complained about not having enough time to get everything done— therefore, they were more likely to take shortcuts, such as driving to nearby errands instead of walking.

TORCH CALORIES

Just 10 minutes of moderate exercise dials up your metabolism for an hour or longer, reports the journal *Science Translational Medicine*. Researchers found that levels of molecules involved in calorie burning changed significantly an hour after a 10-minute treadmill test—in some cases doubling among the fittest test subjects.

LOWER ANXIETY

Studies suggest that small doses of regular exercise—we're talking 10 to 20 minutes at a time—can result in temporary mood improvement or anxiety reduction. Exercise raises levels of serotonin, a feel-good hormone, while reducing your heart rate, blood pressure, and stress hormone levels.

STRONGER FUTURE

A little exercise goes a long way when it comes to protecting your bones and heart down the road. Research shows that just 10 minutes of high-impact exercise (like plyometrics) three times a week can boost women's bone strength—a critical factor in staving off osteoporosis later in life. And doing just 30 minutes of weight training a week is linked to a 23 percent decrease in heart disease risk, according to Harvard researchers.

ANOTHER REASON TO STICK WITH IT

If you take a few weeks or months (or even years!) off from exercise, you will most likely huff and puff and feel achy as your body gets back into the swing of things. But if you establish a history of regular exercise, your pain will be a lot more manageable. That's because any sweat equity you invest forges a cardiovascular and strength blueprint that helps you make gains faster and become less prone to soreness and injury.

It's a phenomenon aptly called "muscle memory." When you learn something new, whether it's how to do a split squat or snowboard, your brain fires up nerves that signal the muscle fibers to kick in. Once your muscle fibers get the memo from your brain to move, they start sending messages back. Movement activates sensors (called proprioceptors) in your muscles, tendons, and joints that constantly give feedback to your central nervous system about where your body is in space, so it knows what muscles to fire next. It's a continuous feedback loop from your brain to your muscles and back. Over time, your brain creates pathways through your central nervous system, and movements become automatic. That's why even if you haven't hopped on a bike in years, your body remembers what to do.

Think of it like a health savings account: The earlier you start and the more you build, the better off you'll be later in life—even if your deposits stall for a while. Case in point: Ohio University researchers put a group of women on a 2-day-a-week strength-training program for 20 weeks, and then let them lounge around for 8 months. When the researchers called these women back to the gym along with a group of women who'd never lifted before, they found that the previously trained group had retained most of their muscle memory. When they started pumping iron again, these women made gains more rapidly than the women with no history of strength training.

QUICK TIPS:
SELF-CARE

9 **Sweat away brain pain.** Moderate aerobic exercise can ease tension headaches by triggering the release of pain-relieving endorphins, according to research in *Current Pain and Headache Reports.* Try 20 minutes of brisk walking or cycling, and drink plenty of water—dehydration can make head pounders even worse, say study authors.

10 **Take a walk.** People who took a brisk 15-minute walk ate 46 percent less chocolate afterward compared to people who sat quietly for 15 minutes.

11 **Keep it moving.** The dangers of sitting too much may drill all the way down to your DNA: Australian researchers sampled thigh muscles from people who sat constantly and those who took 2-minute walking breaks every 20 minutes. The latter group showed positive changes in 75 genes, including one involved with new muscle growth and the destruction of free radicals.

12 **Aim for 150 minutes per week.** Getting in your 150 minutes of weekly exercise could negate the risk for death by cancer that moderate drinking presents, one study found.

13 **Exercise yourself happy.** According to a study published in *Medicine & Science in Sports & Exercise,* women who met the National Activity Guidelines had a 48 percent lower risk of depressive symptoms compared to inactive women. Exercise lifts levels of serotonin, the same feel-good brain chemical made more accessible by some antidepressants.

14 **Join a program.** Forty-seven percent of women in a weight-loss program no longer met criteria for clinical depression after 1 year—without therapy or meds.

QUICK TIPS:
SELF-CARE *(cont.)*

15 **Get a post-gym boost.** For an extra shot of self-discipline, hit the gym. A quick, moderately intense workout could boost self-control immediately afterward, according to a research review published in the *British Journal of Sports Medicine.* Exercise seems to increase blood and oxygen flow to areas of the brain responsible for such skills as restraint and focus. An easy jog for as little as 20 minutes can do the trick.

16 **Lift away diabetes risk.** Research in *PLOS Medicine* suggests that strength training for at least an hour a week slashes a woman's risk of developing type 2 diabetes by 28 percent.

17 **Go your own way.** You love running, but your friend swears by yoga? You both win. When study participants logged at least three weekly 30-minute sessions of running or yoga, both groups saw a dramatic drop in resting heart rate, depression, and perceived stress levels compared to the sedentary group.

18 **See the light.** In a study, people who had the majority of their natural light exposure in the a.m. had lower BMIs compared with those whose rays came later in the day. Getting light in the early hours can alter satiety hormones and may help regulate your circadian rhythms, which could help ward off weight gain, say study authors. Try to move your morning workouts outdoors when you can, raise your shades as soon as your alarm goes off, or eat breakfast next to a light box with a brightness of more than 500 lux, which researchers say can mimic the sun's power.

EVERY DAY IS A NEW BEGINNING. TREAT IT THAT WAY.

FITNESS FIX

3

Rethinking Your Relationship with Food & Fitness

OUT OF ALL THE fitness myths, one of the most destructive is that you need to live at the gym to sculpt a strong, healthy body. That's because it has a polarizing effect: Some women reject working out altogether, either because they're too daunted to get started or they've tried and failed; others unknowingly push themselves beyond the point of progress. Women tell me all the time—with great pride—about their back-to-back spin classes or the boot camp where they did hundreds of crunches and burpees, or how they knocked out a 10-mile run just for the heck of it.

Impressive? Absolutely. Effective? That depends on your goal. More often than not, these lengthy routines don't have a direct correlation to physical changes. And super-active women are still griping about stubborn belly fat, wishing to lose those last 5 pounds. The problem isn't with their effort, it's with their approach. (In fact, research shows that 97 percent of dieters regain the weight they lost, and experts suspect that the likely cause is their workout method.)

Some of it can be attributed to this: For almost two decades, we've been hearing the seductive call of the "fat-burning zone," in which you burn a greater percentage of fat calories. And we've been told you get there by doing moderate—not hard—exercise. But it's not that simple. When you exercise at 60 to 70 percent of your maximum heart rate, in that so-called zone, you burn fewer calories per minute during and after your workout. That's why if you look inside any gym here in America, you'll see rows of people sweating it out on treadmills (or ellipticals, stair steppers, or stationary bikes)—and if you stop in again months later, many of those same people won't look that much slimmer, despite the countless hours they've spent in those crowded cardio rooms.

Picture your physical activity level on a spectrum. At one end is the effortless kind, like sitting at your desk or walking to a meeting. When you're not exerting yourself, your body actually burns a higher percentage of calories from fat than it does when you're active. That's partly why the fat-burning zone was so appealing—it sounds awesome. But, of course, that doesn't mean sitting at your desk or wandering the halls at work will shrink your hips faster than doing jumping jacks or running a sprint.

Now, toward the other end of the activity spectrum is a super-intense workout that sends your heart rate way beyond the classic fat-burning zone. At this point, your body needs quick energy, so it starts burning less flab and turns instead to carbohydrates, which enter the bloodstream faster than fat does. The upside: The harder you work, the more calories you burn. At your max effort, experts estimate that you could be burning 20 to 30 calories a minute. And it's the total number of calories you burn that actually blasts body fat.

Besides burning more calories per minute, high-intensity exercise unleashes a flood of hormones, including epinephrine, that helps your body burn calories even when you're not working out. Case in point: People who cycled at a high intensity for 20 minutes torched more calories for hours after their workouts than they did after cycling at a low intensity for 30 to 60 minutes, according to a study reported in *Medicine & Science in Sports & Exercise*. You won't get those benefits from exercising in the classic fat-burning zone.

TIME TO LIFT WEIGHTS

So if you think cardio is the key to big results, this is definitely a chapter you want to read carefully. There really is no simpler way to say it: Strength training may be the single most efficient way to score a slimmer, sexier body. One study in the journal *Obesity* found that if you're going to add 20 minutes to any routine, you should make it weights rather than running. Participants who used that time to lift weights whittled twice as many centimeters from their waistlines as those who opted for aerobics. It also gives you an edge over belly fat, stress, heart disease, and cancer—and the list goes on and on. In fact, a number of respected fitness pros suggest ditching traditional cardio altogether. So why is it that, according to the *American Journal of Public Health,* only 16 percent of women meet the government's guideline for two or more strength-training sessions a week? Probably because we can't seem to shake these prevalent myths.

CARDIO BURNS MORE CALORIES

For ages, many experts have said that, calorie for calorie, aerobic exercise burns more calories than pumping iron. Not to mention, it feels true; not every trip to the weight room leaves you drenched and out of breath like a killer spin class (especially given that lifting newbies tend to have lower overall intensity, usually because they're hesitant). But it turns out that strength training has more calorie-torching potential than it was originally given credit for. Researchers at the University of Southern Maine found that completing a circuit of eight moves (which takes about 8 minutes) can expend 159 to 231 calories. This is about what you'd burn if you ran at a 10-mile-per-hour pace for the same duration.

In fact, the term cardio shouldn't be limited to only aerobic exercise: A study at the University of Hawaii found that circuit training with weights raises your heart rate 15 beats per minute higher than if you ran at 60 to 70 percent of your max heart rate. The circuit approach provides cardiovascular benefits similar to those of aerobic exercise while strengthening your muscles—so you save time without sacrificing results.

But here's where lifting really shines: Unlike aerobic exercise, the researchers found that a total-body workout with just three big-muscle moves raised participants' metabolisms for 39 hours afterward. Translation: Your body will continue to burn calories at a faster rate long after you've kicked off your sneakers. Sweet deal, right?

YOU CAN OUTRUN BELLY FAT

This one's not even close: Weight training torches body fat better than hours of cardio, plain and simple. In a study at the University of Alabama at Birmingham, one group of dieters lifted three times a week and another did aerobic exercise for the same amount of time. Both groups consumed the same number of calories, and both shed the same amount of weight (26 pounds). But those who pumped iron dropped 100 percent fat, whereas the cardio group lost 92 percent fat and 8 percent muscle. Here's why this matters: Muscle loss may drop your scale weight, but it doesn't improve your reflection in the mirror, and it makes you more likely to gain back the flab you lost. But if you strength-train while you diet, you'll build fat-fighting lean muscle mass and burn more fat. Experts estimate that for every 3 pounds of muscle you build, you can burn an extra 120 calories a day—just vegging—because muscle takes more energy to sustain. Over the course of a year, that's about 10 pounds of fat—without spending more time in the gym or changing your diet.

AEROBIC EXERCISE KEEPS YOUR HEART HEALTHY

Okay, yes, that's true, but cardio isn't the only way to get your blood pumping. Cardio improves heart health (lowering resting heart rate, increasing work output), cholesterol levels, and your body's ability to metabolize sugars, which is why you need it even if weight loss isn't one of your goals. But many women associate cardio with only things like running, swimming, biking, and brisk walking—what experts typically label "aerobic exercise." That's a limiting definition. Cardio—aka cardiovascular exercise—is any activity that strengthens your heart and improves the function of your cardiovascular system. To do this, major muscle groups need to contract repeatedly enough to elevate your heart rate to a target level. (Some experts give a general ballpark of at least 50 percent of your max, or about 100 beats per minute.)

That means the umbrella of cardiovascular exercise includes both aerobic and anaerobic workouts—aerobic being a light to moderate sustained effort that needs oxygen to help fuel your muscles, and anaerobic being a typically shorter but tougher effort—which means a 30-minute treadmill jog at lunch counts, but so does a kettlebell circuit. In fact, researchers at the University of Michigan found that people who did three total-body weight workouts a week for 2 months decreased their diastolic blood pressure (the bottom number) by an average of eight points. That's enough to reduce your risk of a stroke by 40 percent and your chance of a heart attack by 15 percent.

University of South Carolina researchers determined that total-body strength is linked to a lower risk of death from cardiovascular disease and cancer. Similarly, other scientists found that being strong during middle age is associated with "exceptional survival," defined as living to the age of 85 without developing a major disease.

LIFTING MAKES YOU BULKY

Every day I receive pitches and reviews for new workout methods that create "long and lean muscles." I hear ladies say they don't lift because they're looking to get "toned," not "bulky." We even use it in the magazine as a way of describing the overall aesthetic many of our readers are trying to achieve.

But here's some news that might disappoint a lot of women—and even more trainers who play into the female fear of looking like the Hulk: Muscles, by definition, are lean, and their length is set once your body is mature. No workout can make them leaner, and, outside of surgery, there is not much that can permanently alter their length. In fact, there are only two ways that muscle can change its appearance: It can get bigger or get smaller.

This battle of toning versus bulking actually has nothing to do with the muscles themselves—it comes down to your overall body fat. This idea of looking toned is often an attempt to describe a body with a low enough body fat percentage to reveal muscle definition. When you build muscle but don't attack the body fat that lies on top of it, you may feel bigger or heavier. Conversely, methods like Pilates and yoga typically don't use the same level of resistance, which may mean you're not building as much muscle; so even if your body fat percentage remains the same, you at least don't feel like you're getting denser. At the same time, many of these routines help improve posture, which can give the appearance that you are, in fact, "longer and leaner."

These light-resistance methods can actually sabotage your goals in the long run, though. Research shows that between the ages of 30 and 50, you'll likely lose 10 percent of your body's total muscle. Worse yet, it's likely to be

FOR THE RECORD

Another myth I hear people repeating all the time: Muscle can turn into fat. Let's clear this one up. These are two totally different types of tissue, so even if you slack off, that hard-earned muscle won't turn into fat. With lack of use, muscle cells atrophy. If they shrink to a certain size, they undergo apoptosis (or die). They don't miraculously transform into fat cells. That's not to say there's not a relationship between the two: If you lose muscle mass, you'll burn fewer calories per day, and if your calorie intake remains the same, the excess food energy that is not burned can be stored as fat.

replaced by fat over time, according to a study in the *American Journal of Clinical Nutrition*. Even participants who maintained their body weight for up to 38 years lost 3 pounds of muscle and added 3 pounds of fat every decade.

Why does that matter? Because even if their body weight remained the same, their pants size likely didn't. Not only does lean muscle mass help stoke your internal calorie burner, but it also actually takes up 18 percent less space than 1 pound of fat. So to recap: Building lean muscle mass through strength training is the real secret to revealing a leaner, more toned body.

TO RUN BETTER, YOU MUST RUN MORE

Practice makes perfect, right? Turns out, extra pavement pounding isn't the only—or necessarily the most effective—strategy. A review of studies in the *Journal of Strength and Conditioning Research* found that runners who did resistance-training exercises 2 or 3 days a week, in addition to their weekly cardio regimens, increased their leg strength and enhanced their endurance—two things that improve performance and contribute to weight loss.

Lifting can also keep you injury free: A study in the journal *Clinical Biomechanics* found that female runners who did 6 weeks of lower-body exercises improved their leg strength, particularly in their hips—a common source of pain and injury for runners.

YOU NEED A PRICEY GYM MEMBERSHIP

No costly memberships, no sweaty strangers, no stressing to get there before it closes—it's no big surprise that people with home gyms were 73 percent more likely to be active than those without them. But you don't need a ton of equipment to get into great shape. Here are a few of the best pieces to bring home.

DUMBBELLS / There's nothing glitzy about them, but dumbbells are the single most essential workout tool to keep around. There are literally hundreds of exercises you can do with them. If you can, get at least two pairs (one light, one heavy) so that you can switch them up depending on the exercise.

CHINUP BAR / Bodyweight exercises cover every basic movement—except pulling. Nothing trains you better than classic chinups. You can find a number of at-home, removable options.

FOAM ROLLER / Loosen tight fascia (the connective tissue that surrounds muscles) for improved recovery, better performance, and a more lithe look. There are endless options, from full-length roller to travel size, and even small balls that are perfect for targeting small spots in your back, shoulders, hips, and glutes.

VALSLIDE / These sliding discs increase the friction of almost any surface—turning your hardwood floor, carpet, or tile into a skating rink. The result: Your muscles are under constant tension during every exercise, which boosts the effectiveness. (Find a Valslide workout on page 162.)

STABILITY BALL / It's a great tool for core exercises and can also substitute for a bench in some exercises to increase the difficulty and increase your core activation.

TRX / This suspension trainer leverages your own weight to adjust the resistance of any total-body move. Setup is simple—just flip over a door or around a (sturdy) stair banister—

and it packs into a small bag so you can stash it when you're not using it.

RESISTANCE BANDS / Big ones can make bodyweight squats extra challenging or help with assisted chinups, while smaller bands are some of my favorite tools for waking up the underworked muscles in your hips and butt.

KETTLEBELL / It can be used in the same way as dumbbells, but because of its unique shape, it's even more versatile. (Find the ultimate lean-body kettlebell workout on page 145.)

JUMP ROPE / For just a few bucks you can have a portable, calorie-incinerating tool that's perfect for picking up your heart rate during a warmup or spiking your calorie-burn totals during your workout.

BENCH, STEP, OR BOX / Adjustable benches add variety to free-weight training; a basic cardio step or box can be a great starting point for beginners.

GET COMFY IN THE KITCHEN

One of the best pieces of fitness advice I received early in my job at *Women's Health* was: "You can't out-exercise a bad diet." If there's one thing you pick up from this chapter, it should be that. Why? Even top trainers will tell you that when it comes to losing body fat, it doesn't matter how often, how hard, or how long you work out—nutrition is going to be the key to your success. Building muscle is crucial for increasing definition and boosting your metabolism, but if you want to get serious about getting in shape, you've got to realign your priorities. It's all about the food.

In fact, starting an exercise program for the sole purpose of burning fat or losing weight is counterproductive. Researchers at the University of Minnesota pitted calorie restriction without exercise against cardio workouts with no dietary changes. The diet-only women lost significantly more weight in 8 weeks than those who exercised. But don't cancel your gym membership just yet: The same study found that women lost the most weight when they combined diet and exercise.

One reason your workout may not be working—or at least not as well as you think it is: People grossly overestimate how many calories they burn during exercise, especially when they think it's high-intensity. Estimating calorie output can be an inexact science; it involves factors like age, weight, body temperature, metabolic rate, and hormonal changes (to name a few) that are complicated, difficult to track, and ever-fluctuating. It doesn't help when your boot-camp instructor says that each class blasts 1,000 calories (a total exaggeration) or you check the counters on cardio machines. (Ellipticals have been reported to overestimate expenditure by 42 percent.)

A bigger problem: Women sometimes use these assumptions about their workouts to make decisions on how they eat for the rest of the day. Translation: When you believe your workout just torched 800 calories, you feel less guilty about the whip on your Frappuccino or those cookies after dinner.

Moderately active women typically need about 1,800 to 2,200 calories a day to maintain their weight. To drop pounds, you'll need to shave anywhere from 250 to 500 calories a day from that total. Seems simple, right? Not quite. According to a study published in the *Journal of Sports Medicine and Physical Fitness,* college students consumed up to three times more calories than they burned during their last workout. Researchers believe that following exercise, people may be less mindful of what they're putting into their mouths. Not only that, but after an intense workout session many women also tend to be less active throughout the rest of the day (by, say, not taking the stairs or spending more downtime on the couch). Researchers at the University of South Carolina found that women burned 70 fewer calories during the day after doing a hard workout compared with days they didn't hit the gym.

That last part is crucial: Think of all the opportunities you have to be active in between workouts—taking the stairs instead of the elevator, walking across the office instead of sending an e-mail, or riding a bike instead of taking a cab. These on-the-go activities help you sneak in exercise without really even thinking about it.

Mindless, on-the-move eating, however? Yeah, that doesn't help your weight-loss efforts. This is because mobile foods, although convenient, tend to be the ones most laden with fat, sugar, and sodium. Snacks in general have more calories than ever before.

When you stop and think about the food–fitness connection, you can see how Brazilian researchers found that up to 75 percent of weight loss is controlled by diet. That's not to say that your workouts aren't important, but instead that it's time to drop the mindset that your hard-earned sweat can balance out your daily food choices. Focus on the muscle-building, metabolism-revving perks of your workout, rather than making your calorie-burn total the primary goal.

HUNGER GAMES

How you feel after working out—exhausted, drained, and possibly ravenous—can reinforce the idea that you burned a ton of calories and your body needs more fuel. (Not to mention that it can make you believe you deserve a treat.) While serious athletes need extra calories to offset their demanding training, the average woman has enough glycogen stored in her muscles and liver to power her through a workout.

That said, a 200-calorie snack (a mix of carbs and protein) during the hour after your workout can help muscle recovery efforts and restore glycogen supplies so you won't reach for candy later. Just remember to figure these calories into your daily count.

QUICK TIPS:
SNACKING

19 **Cut it in half.** A study in the *Journal of the American Dietetic Association* found that people who were given the same snack, either whole or cut into halves, consumed half as much when eating the latter, possibly because they considered only the number of items (not the size of the items) they ate.

20 **Chew a piece of sugarfree gum.** People ate 60 fewer calories worth of sugary snacks later in the day when they chewed sugar-free gum after lunch. A University of Rhode Island study found that chewing stimulates nerves that are connected to the area of the brain responsible for satiety.

21 **Keep it funny.** Watching engaging comedies can help curb mindless snacking, according to *PLOS ONE.* Women downed 52 percent more when viewing a dull program compared with a more entertaining one. Study authors say boredom is one of the strongest motivators in leading people to eat. Go one step further: Curl up with a pre-portioned snack to help prevent overeating.

22 **Don't judge a snack by its wrapper.** According to a study in *Appetite,* participants served themselves 50 percent more of a snack when it had "fitness" on the label—despite the fact that the other food offered had the same amount of fat and calories.

23 **Avoid social media.** People who browsed Facebook for 5 minutes were more likely to choose an unhealthy snack afterward than those who spent the same amount of time scanning a news site. Clicking through friends' walls or photos makes you feel more connected to them and temporarily gives your self-esteem a boost. Unfortunately, this decreases self-control, say study co-authors Keith Wilcox, PhD, of Columbia University and Andrew T. Stephen, PhD, of the University of Pittsburgh. They recommend avoiding social media when you're hungry, since that's when your willpower is already low.

24 Get off to a strong start. To put the kibosh on midnight munchies, eat a high-protein breakfast. In a study, women started their day with either eggs and lean beef or a lower-protein cereal. Having a high-protein morning meal resulted in participants snacking on about 135 fewer after-dinner calories. Protein-rich meals prevent the secretion of the hunger hormone ghrelin and stimulate release of the satiety hormone peptide YY.

25 Beef up your office snacks. After sitting at your desk all morning, you're less likely to burn off carbohydrates. Curb your carb intake and increase the amount of healthy fat you consume in the afternoon by choosing low-fat string cheese or walnuts.

26 Fill up on fruit. When you have an indulgent day of eating, snack on produce. Mice that ate a high-fat, high-sugar diet gained less weight when they received a supplement of fermentable fiber—a type found in many fruits and vegetables. Translation: Adding these foods may help you stay trim, even if you don't cut the junk. The fiber boosts glucose production, which helps you torch more calories, according to researchers.

27 Keep your counters clean. Leave nutritious snacks out instead of storing them in your pantry. Researchers have found that the mere sight of good-for-you food can help you munch less. They suspect the presence of food linked with healthy eating may be a reminder of a long-term goal to lose weight.

YOUR WORKOUTS SHOULD BE A CELEBRATION OF WHAT YOUR BODY CAN DO, NOT A PUNISHMENT FOR WHAT YOU ATE.

FITNESS FIX

4 / Diet Secrets of the Slim & Healthy

LAUNCH INTO PRETTY MUCH any diet plan and you're bound to lose some weight. It's not magic; suddenly, you're not randomly grazing—you're following a meal plan and eating with a purpose, no matter how sound (or unsound) that purpose is. The problem is, your brain is a calorie hog, and it takes an immense amount of concentration to stick to a complicated diet. Not to mention that, from day one, most don't feel sustainable—so you know from the get-go it's a temporary fix. The super-simple principles you'll find throughout this chapter make losing weight doable, not daunting. They may even feel too easy or basic to work, but that's the point. Your results may not show up as quickly as fad diets' do. But while they're not as quick, they're lasting. By trading in your old dieting ways, you'll save time in the long run because you'll be able to sustain these, and therefore maintain your lighter weight. Learn to eat healthy, one meal at a time, by ditching deprivation and shifting to a new way of eating—and say goodbye to your fickle and fluctuating relationship with the scale.

TAKE BABY STEPS TO BETTER

Let's be realistic: You aren't going to trade in potato chips for kale chips, fried chicken for broiled, or ice cream for frozen grapes overnight. And that's why most diets fail you. They often deprive you of foods that your body is accustomed to and replace them with überhealthy choices that sound the alarm to let your brain know you're on a diet—a move that sets you up for out-of-control cravings and, eventually, weight-gain relapse.

Instead of going cold turkey, transition from less healthy eats to better ones in baby steps. For the first week, don't even make it about the food—just focus on drinking six to eight glasses of water a day. Then, during the second week, trade $1/2$ cup of your rice or pasta at dinner for the same amount of vegetables. Then, try ordering your bacon cheeseburger on a bed of lettuce rather than a bun, and so on. The examples below demonstrate how to wean yourself off less-than-ideal grub. Spend 2 to 4 weeks at each stage—the reward system in your brain needs time to adapt. These small moves will build confidence and teach your body to enjoy healthy foods that satisfy hunger—without any frustration or burnout. Success, then, results from targeted efficiency rather than probability.

I promise—after a few weeks you won't be focusing on the changes to your plate, only the ones to your waistline.

BREAKFAST

GOOD	BETTER	BEST
Homemade Blueberry-Yogurt Muffins	**2 Scrambled Eggs, 1 Package of Plain Instant Oatmeal**	**Omelet Wrap**
Going for baked over store-bought immediately boosts the nutrition—plus they have a fraction of the calories and keep the sugar and fat in check.	Eggs are a complete protein, and having them in the morning can kick-start your metabolism. Pairing them with oatmeal's healthy carbs will hold off hunger until lunch.	Use one egg and one egg white to save about 40 calories (compared with two whole eggs), veggies for low-cal fiber, 1 tablespoon of cheese, and a whole wheat wrap. Quick, filling, and delicious—a weight-loss trifecta.

SALAD

GOOD	BETTER	BEST
Romaine with 1 Tablespoon of Creamy Dressing	**Romaine with 1 Tablespoon of Balsamic Vinaigrette**	**Baby Spinach with 1 Tablespoon of Balsamic Vinaigrette**
Romaine packs more antioxidants in its leaves than, say, iceberg lettuce, and sticking to just 1 tablespoon dressing slashes an easy 70 calories.	Don't reach for the fat-free kind: The olive oil in the regular variety contains healthy fats to keep you satisfied longer.	Spinach leaves are full of B vitamins, which may help lower your risk for certain cancers.

CHIPS

GOOD	BETTER	BEST
Baked Potato Chips	**Bean Chips**	**Kale Chips**
It's a step in the right direction, with 40 fewer calories and 8 fewer grams of fat per serving compared to regular potato chips. But white spuds aren't exactly a weight-loss superfood.	Many kinds have more calories than baked chips, but they're also packed with about 4 grams of protein and 5 grams of fiber per serving, so they're more filling.	These babies pack fiber, vitamin A, calcium for bone strength, vitamin C to grow cells, and vitamin K, which may help bone growth. They're simple to make at home, too (find a few recipes on page 244).

CHICKEN

GOOD	BETTER	BEST
Baked Chicken with Barbecue Sauce	**Chicken Parmesan**	**Grilled or Baked Herb-Crusted Chicken**
You ditch the dangerous saturated fat found in the crunchy coating of fried chicken—which is a plus—but most finger-licking sauces are loaded with sugar and salt.	Little to no sugar here, but keep the shredded cheese to 4 teaspoons max to control the fat and calories.	Compared to its fried counterpart, where you started, this flavor-packed alternative can save you nearly 7 grams of saturated fat and 200 calories.

KEEP IT CONSISTENT

Make sure your approach to eating is one you can stick with. Ask yourself, "Can I see myself eating like this forever?" If the answer is no, you need to change your approach. You should think of this as a permanent lifestyle shift.

And consistency doesn't just mean Monday through Friday, either. Researchers have found that people who eat consistently day to day are one and a half times more likely to maintain their weight loss than those who diet only on weekdays. For most people, weekends mean relaxing their diet or indulging in a few splurges, and a study in the *Journal of Public Policy & Marketing* found that adults scarf down, on average, 419 extra calories each weekend.

At the same time, it's important to remember that one meal doesn't define your diet—and it doesn't mean you've failed or fallen off the wagon. So maybe you couldn't stop yourself from polishing off the entire caramel sundae (that came after the spinach dip and chicken quesadillas), but that's no reason to give up entirely. Instead, think of it this way: Every meal is a chance to start over and do it right. Follow up a fall from nutritional grace with healthy choices the next five times you eat. This means you'll be eating right more than 80 percent of the time. It's what you eat the majority of the time that has an impact on your waistline.

Case in point: One study found that the most successful dieters practiced simple habits (like putting down their fork between bites, eating a hot breakfast within an hour of waking up, and portioning out food before digging in) a minimum of 25 days per month. Just by establishing more consistent healthy-eating habits, the group dropped an average of 2 pounds per month.

TAKE CONTROL

Don't rely on hope and prayers to get the body you want. Investing just an hour or two on the weekend to get a jump start on preparing your meals for the week (cutting veggies, making marinades) will save you time and pounds in the long run. Creating a "menu" each week—say, grilled chicken with roasted vegetables on Monday night, yogurt with fresh fruit and granola for Tuesday's breakfast, and so on—creates a confident path to success. A survey by the Centers for Disease Control and Prevention found that almost 40 percent of people who lost a significant amount of weight and kept it off planned their weekly meals. When you don't map out your meals, you're too tempted to grab whatever's nearby, which is often high-calorie junk.

If arranging every meal feels too rigid, map out a list of potential options for your meals and snacks based on the foods you have available, instead. This will give you the flexibility to choose based on your tastes at the time, but the hard part (thinking of something to make) will already be out of the way. According to Dutch researchers, thinking about snacks and meals can actually help you stay lean. The study found that when asked questions like, "What will you do if you get hungry 2 hours before your next meal?" thinner participants were better able to give healthy responses like, "eat a handful of nuts."

Planning ahead can also help prevent slipups. How many times have you actually driven to the store late at night to pick up a pint of ice cream? Now, compare that to how many times you've raided your fridge. You're more likely to give in to a craving when the object you desire is close at hand. Simple solution: Make sure it's not. Do your meal brainstorming before you head to the grocery store and make a list of the ingredients you need for the upcoming week; sticking to just what you have outlined can help you skip impulse items, and you'll get in and out of the store quicker.

FIND YOUR OWN FREQUENCY

Around the turn of the millennium, research began to sing the benefits of eating more frequently (as opposed to sticking to three main meals). The "graze, don't gorge" philosophy is based on the idea that having frequent small meals

'TIS THE SEASON FOR TEMPTATION

There's a reason we're such suckers for holiday treats: Decades of research show that items we perceive as being in limited supply seem more desirable to us than items we see all year round. Give yourself a limited allotment of your favorite holiday treat (like Starbucks Peppermint Mochas or McDonald's Shamrock Shakes) and stick to it.

keeps your blood sugar steady, your metabolism ramped up, and your appetite in check. A big part of the logic is that going too long between meals—or skipping them completely—may lead to overeating later. It could even explain why women who skipped meals lost about 8 pounds less than those who ate more consistently, according to a study in the *Journal of the Academy of Nutrition and Dietetics*.

Here's the thing: Other research shows a link between obesity and eating more than three times a day, most notably in women. After all, more frequent noshing means more opportunities to overeat. Plus, having to constantly think about what you're going to eat can be stressful, especially for emotional eaters.

The verdict: The mini-meal approach doesn't work for everyone—and it doesn't have to. You'll eat healthiest if you eat your way—meaning, if you prefer substantial meals fewer times a day, there's no reason to force yourself to do the opposite. In yet another study, from Warwick Medical School in the United Kingdom, women saw the same daily calorie burn whether they tucked into two large meals or five small ones. Once you find an eating pattern that keeps you satisfied, stick with it. Changing the pattern of when you eat may affect hunger-hormone levels because your brain becomes used to eating at certain times, and a shift could throw it off, researchers say.

EAT FOOD YOU ACTUALLY LIKE

If eating nothing but raw foods, or locally sourced meat, or cabbage soup sounds enjoyable to you—go for it. But for the vast majority of people, these aren't maintainable eating options, they're diets. To be sustainable, you have to actually like, not just tolerate, the food you're being told to eat, just like with exercising. If you don't, you start off knowing it's going to be a short-term gig, which could make you throw in the towel even sooner.

But while a strict program can be a great tool for resetting your eating habits, if it's not tailored to your schedule, budget, and personal preferences, it will eventually fail. That's not to say you won't see any results. In fact, any time you completely eliminate something from your diet—say, gluten, sugar, processed foods, or booze—you tend to shed some weight. It's partly what bolsters the allure of fad diets—people "prove" they are effective by getting results.

However, for a diet plan to work in the long run, it has to be meaningful to you. Does a particular diet call for a list of organic or fresh foods that cost more than your weekly take-home pay or that might spoil before you can eat them? Find frozen varieties for a fraction of the cost; they will keep if you're only cooking for one. Does your French-inspired meal plan call for blue cheese on everything, but you despise the taste? Switch to mozzarella, or Swiss, or feta cheese. Do you crave carbs every day, despite your resolve to stick to Atkins? The truth is, aside from medical or ethical reasons, there's no real payoff to nixing entire food groups. Instead of dropping carbohydrates, for example, refigure your approach to focus on making better choices on the sources (say, by swapping cheesy potatoes au gratin for a baked sweet potato or roasted fingerlings).

When it comes to weight loss, your total calorie intake is what matters the most. If you eat fewer calories than you burn on a cabbage-soup diet, you will lose weight. Likewise, if you eat more than you burn, the surplus can lead to weight gain, regardless of what foods those calories come from. By making meal decisions based on your tastes and preferences rather than on what your friend eats or the latest fad diet, you'll feel more satisfied by every meal.

SIZE EVERYTHING UP

While variables like meal timing and the division of macronutrients are always hot topics to debate, there's one thing everyone should be able to agree on: Size matters.

Our portion-control meter doesn't register like it used to; in today's super-sized society, our measure of a "just right" serving is far larger than it was just 30 years ago. This has had an impact on our ability to eye up proper portions. According to Purdue University researchers, the biggest problem with our snacking habits is that our between-meal bites have taken on actual meal–size proportions, and our actual meals have become feasts by comparison. It's not even because we're hungry: In one study, Pennsylvania State University researchers found that subjects ate 30 percent more food when presented with bigger portions, yet their perceived fullness didn't change.

Fad diets and nixed food groups have also contributed. Say you're following a sort of low-carb, high-protein diet where 40 percent of your daily calories come from protein, 40 percent from dietary fat, and 20 percent from carbohydrates. In this scenario, you can eat plenty of peanut butter or bacon (or peanut butter and bacon, a combination that creates one of my dad's favorite sandwiches) without gaining weight because of the overall calorie split. But when you veer off course or ditch the diet completely, you have to readjust those percentages. If you continue to eat the same portion sizes, but now with bread, you're likely getting more calories than you need, which can lead to weight gain.

There's another sneaky portion problem that you're likely not keeping a close eye on. Women often tell me (with great pride) about their healthy meal choices: They start their day with Greek yogurt with fresh berries and granola; snack on an apple with peanut butter or carrots with hummus; their lunchtime salad is topped with avocado, walnuts, hard-cooked eggs, and feta cheese; dinners are a well-balanced mix of brown rice, chicken, and roasted veggies. That all sounds fantastic, right? Of course, but there's a crucial question that needs to be asked, especially if these women are still struggling to hit their goal weights: "How much?" While the food choices are spot on, it is possible to have too much of a good thing.

TRACK FEELINGS, NOT CALORIES

Our tracking-app age has intensified this idea that a "calorie is a calorie"—that weight loss isn't really about what you eat, but how many calories you eat. As long as your weight-loss app says you came in under your daily caloric totals, it doesn't matter if you had two candy bars for lunch. While counting each and every calorie may help keep your intake in check, it can also take up way too much of your time and make you feel crazy. Not to mention that it's not always accurate: According to researchers from Tufts University, restaurants underreport the number of calories in their food by 18 percent on average. So if you're eating what you think is a 600-calorie burger, there's a good chance it's actually north of 700 calories.

For a minute, consider the irony of the whole eat-like-a-caveman approach to the Paleo Diet: Our prehistoric ancestors didn't diet. They didn't stress over contradicting rules like carbs versus no carbs, breakfast versus no breakfast. They didn't judge the food they were eating or worry about how many calories it contained. Their approach was much more intuitive: Find quality food (day-old meat or half-rotted vegetables wouldn't do), and eat enough to have energy to get through the tasks of the day.

If more of us adopted their mindset rather than their menu, we might have better results—and, I'd argue, feel a lot less overwhelmed and bogged down by healthy eating. Researchers at the University of Texas at Austin found that women lost more weight by learning behavior-change strategies and minding their hunger cues than by fixating on external cues (like an empty plate) or diet rules (like eating a certain number of calories).

PRACTICE MAKES PERMANENT

People who learned skills for maintaining a steady weight before starting a diet were more likely to keep pounds off than those who dieted right away, according to a study in the *Journal of Consulting and Clinical Psychology.* Participants who mastered maintenance habits—like finding tasty low-cal swaps for high-cal foods and eating mindfully—regained only 3 pounds after a year, compared with 7 pounds among the diet-first group. Thinking things through when you're starting out harnesses your enthusiasm and channels it into keeping weight off—the part of dieting people struggle with most, say the study authors.

Try a little experiment: For 1 week, take a break from the numbers and, instead, keep track of when you eat and how you feel. Look for patterns. Do you always hit up your coworker's candy jar after a tough meeting? Do you graze before dinner out of boredom? Do you always crave ice cream after seeing a Dairy Queen commercial? Identifying and working to change these habits can help you slim down in the long run.

LOSE THE LABELS

You thought I was talking about the ones on packaged foods, didn't you? That works, too, but it's not what I'm referring to. When it comes to nutrition, everyone today seems to be looking for a good guy and a bad guy. But putting a mental safety lock on "bad" foods doesn't guarantee results. According to a study in the *American Journal of Clinical Nutrition,* participants who restricted their junk-food intake shed the same amount of weight as those who didn't. The researchers found that subjects who deprived themselves still splurged—just on other grub. It can also actually make you crave the off-limits food more: Women who suppressed thoughts about chocolate craved it more—and ate more when they gave in.

Even your positive association with healthy foods can expand your waist-line: Turns out, the fewer calories you think a food has, the more of it you tend to eat. (In one study, people were shown a bowl of chili alone and another bowl next to a plate of greens—and they underestimated the number of calories in the chili with the salad.) Experts refer to it as the "health halo" effect, and manufacturers and restaurants use it against you by making foods sound healthier: A study in the *Journal of Consumer Research* found that people, particularly those with a history of dieting, tended to consume more when a food had a description like "fruit chews" than when the identical nosh was called "candy chews."

And then there are the ever-confusing food wars: It feels like every other month a different staple is being brought back from the hall of shame—or being cast into it. Think one of these is off-limits? Consider the counterevidence.

GLUTEN

For those with a gluten intolerance, dropping the protein found in wheat, rye, and barley is necessary. If you try going sans gluten for a few weeks and notice no substantial difference, there's likely no need to drop it completely.

RED MEAT

Red meat may be higher in calories, fat, and saturated fat than, say, chicken or fish, but there are plenty of diet-friendly cuts—usually called round, tender-loin, or roast. Look for cuts labeled at least 95 percent lean, and keep your portion to 3 or 4 ounces—roughly the size of a smartphone.

DAIRY

Cutting back on the amount of dairy you eat can signal your body to make more fat cells, according to a study in the *American Journal of Clinical Nutrition.* When you don't have enough calcium in your body, it tries to hold on to what's there. This triggers the release of a compound called calcitriol, which increases the production of fat cells.

CARBOHYDRATES

People who make rice part of their daily diet weigh less than those who don't regularly eat the grain, according to a study in Nutrition Today. Besides being packed with belly-filling fiber and valuable nutrients, rice is also more likely to be paired with veggies and lean protein (think stir-fries and sushi) than fatty dishes such as pizza.

EGGS

The incredible, edible egg is actually an excellent, affordable source of protein and B vitamins, and it may help you lose weight. A study in the *International Journal of Obesity* found that dieters who consumed two eggs for breakfast each day lost significantly more weight than those who consumed bagels.

FAT

Fat in any form packs more than twice the amount of calories as protein and carbs. A study published in the *New England Journal of Medicine* found that a diet high in healthy fats is superior to a low-fat diet, both in terms of weight loss and overall health benefits. Fat is filling and adds flavor to your meals—both of which help you avoid feeling deprived. But the source matters: Think nuts, salmon, avocados, and olive oil. Watch the portions: People often eat too much. Olive oil is the number one offender: 1 cup has close to 2,000 calories, and unless you're a stickler for measuring, it's easy to pour on more than the proper 2-teaspoon serving.

SNACK SMARTER

While they are meant to be small bites to keep hunger at bay between meals, today roughly one-quarter of the calories in the American diet come from snacks, according to a study published in the *Journal of Nutrition*.

And snack-size packaging, which supposedly was introduced to help manage our portions, may only make matters worse. Researchers found that dieters inhaled significantly more calories from mini packs of cookies than from standard-size ones. When you finish one bag and still aren't satisfied (the portions are really small, after all), you dig into another—and then another.

Homemade servings are not likely to trigger the same overeating as store-bought packs because the size of the food isn't deceptively smaller—the amount is limited, but to a portion that satisfies you. Reframe your definition of snacks from treats to a mini meal—like a packet of instant oatmeal with a few table-spoons of slivered almonds instead of a candy bar. It may also help to think about what "category" a snack falls into: Is it an All You Can Eat? A Take It Slow? Or a Proceed with Caution? Use these examples as a guide.

ALL YOU CAN EAT

Filling, low-cal treats you don't need to limit: air-popped popcorn; raw veggies (jicama, sugar snap peas, and cherry tomatoes); steamed artichoke (dip in a warm mixture of fat-free plain Greek yogurt and Dijon mustard); fresh ber-ries; cucumber slices marinated in rice wine vinegar and topped with chopped red onions.

TAKE IT SLOW

Enjoy these healthy snacks in mindful moderation: one hard-cooked egg dusted with sea salt and black pepper (70 calories); a 1-ounce chunk of Parme-san (110 calories); three slices of turkey breast wrapped in lettuce, with a little mustard (70 calories).

PROCEED WITH CAUTION

Portion control is key with these nutritious but high-cal options: half an avo-cado with lemon and sea salt (160 calories); ¼ cup of raisins or other dried fruit (123 calories); about 15 nuts or 1 tablespoon of all-natural nut butter (100 calo-ries); 2 tablespoons of hummus (50 calories).

SLOW IT DOWN

Dutch researchers found that big bites and fast chewing can lead to overeating. Participants who chewed larger bites of food for 3 seconds consumed 52 percent more food before feeling full than those who chewed small bites for 9 seconds. The reason: Tasting food for a longer period of time (no matter how much of it) signals your brain to make you feel full sooner. But it can take up to 10 minutes for your brain to get the message that your stomach is full. If you tend to inhale your food, you run the risk of stuffing yourself before realizing you're satiated.

The key to avoiding this button-popping feeling of regret is to eat before you're completely starving (like, say, a 6 on a hunger scale that goes to 10) and spend 20 to 30 minutes on a meal. This is long enough to get that satiety signal, but not so long that you'll be tempted to go for a second helping. And be particularly mindful during dessert: Levels of certain chemicals rise when people eat their favorite foods, reports the *Journal of Clinical Endocrinology & Metabolism,* indicating that the food may turn on the brain's reward system, which overrides signals that you've had enough.

THE SLIMMING POWER OF YOGA

Being a Downward Dog devotee might help you eat less. A study in the *Journal of the American Dietetic Association* found that yoga practitioners tend to eat "mindfully," noshing when hungry and stopping when full. Not so for non-yogis: Even if they exercise daily, they often eat for emotional reasons and past the point of satiety. Yoga helps teach calmness in the face of discomfort, which may make it easier to, say, pass up that slice of cake.

QUICK TIPS: MEALTIME

28 **Make a plan.** Planning ahead doesn't just apply to your at-home meals. When you're eating out, it's almost more crucial to have a plan. Look up the restaurant's menu before you get there to identify a few potential options.

29 **Bypass the bread.** Order a soup or salad as a starter and bypass the bread basket: Researchers found that people eat 47 percent more of a food when they start their meal with it.

30 **Slim down your java.** Use this calorie-cutting lingo at your local coffee shop: *"Hold the whip"* (no whipped cream, cutting anywhere from 50 to 110 calories); *"nonfat"* (replace whole or 2% with fat-free milk); *"sugar-free syrup"* (use instead of regular syrup and save up to 150 calories a drink); *"skinny"* (your drink will be made with sugar-free syrup and fat-free milk).

31 **Order with caution.** Which dinner would you pick off a menu: dumplings or pillowy, fresh, hand-made gnocchi? Yeah, the gnocchi, right? According to research published in the *International Journal of Hospitality Management,* people are 28 percent more likely to order menu items displayed with tantalizing descriptions—which are often the least-healthy choices. Avoid the unintentional indulgence by asking your waiter for recommendations on some of their lighter dishes.

32 **Take your sauces on the side.** When ordering at restaurants like Chipotle, ask for any and all high-calorie add-ons—such as guac, cheese, and sour cream—on the side. Restaurants can easily serve up two to three times the recommended serving size when eyeballing portions. Keeping all your "extras" to a single small plastic cup (like the one your extra guac comes in) will help you keep calories under control.

33 **Keep a tab.** Between the drinks and the bar

food, you could easily put away 1,000 calories at happy hour. Alcohol stimulates your appetite and lowers your inhibitions, so you typically end up caving to cravings—or just eating whatever's around you. The fix: Decide how many drinks you'll have ahead of time, and save a bottle cap, lime wedge, or swizzle stick from each. Studies have found that people tend to consume less when they have a physical reminder of how much they've already had.

34 **Sip smarter.** Anything served in a bottle will help you avoid bartender overpours. Most wines and light beers have 100 to 125 calories per serving; if you want something stronger, try a Manhattan (130 calories), mojito (150), or vodka tonic (170).

35 **Manage movie theater munchies.** If you're busy gazing at Ryan Gosling on the big screen, you're not focused on what you're eating. Sit down with a supersize popcorn, and before you

know it, you've eaten hundreds of calories. (That's no exaggeration: A *Consumer Reports* study found that the largest-size plain popcorn can have 1,269 calories and 81 grams of fat.) The best solution? Control what you put in front of you. At the concession stand, choose the smallest serving size available (researchers found that people tend to eat much more from large containers). Or sneak in your own healthy snack, like homemade trail mix.

36 **Make it Insta-worthy.** Cornell University research shows that eating satisfaction is derived from the flavor intensity and visual impact of a meal, not necessarily the amount served. Kick your food up a notch with spices, which add flavor without adding calories and fat.

37 **Downsize your dishes.** People take less food when they use smaller serving dishes and tall, narrow glasses instead of short, wide ones, a study showed. In another

QUICK TIPS:
MEALTIME *(cont.)*

study, people guessed they were getting 10 percent more food when it was served on a wide-rimmed plate compared to one without a rim.

38 **Prevent overpouring.** Resist filling your bowl to the brim. Serving sizes vary among cereals (for example, a serving of plain Cheerios is 1 cup, while a serving of Honey Nut Cheerios is ¾ cup), and our serving bowls are often much larger than we realize. Get an accurate visual reference by measuring out one serving into your bowl the first time you eat the cereal.

39 **Mind your manners.** People who eat with napkins in their laps tend to have lower body mass indexes.

THOUGHTS BECOME ACTIONS. WHERE WILL YOUR THOUGHTS LEAD YOU?

FITNESS FIX

5 / Workout Secrets of the Super Fit

LIKE WITH A NEW diet, when you launch into a new workout routine you're bound to see—and feel—some progress. The problem is, when you stop seeing results from your workouts, which, for many, can happen around the 6- to 8-week mark, your first instinct may be to stay on the treadmill or elliptical longer or to add a hundred crunches to the end of every workout. But tacking on a few extra minutes won't rescue you from a plateau. The reason: As your body adapts to a particular workout, it becomes more efficient and uses less energy (that is, you burn fewer calories). Just like lifelong healthy eaters, people who seem to always be fit also follow a pretty consistent set of "rules." Their big secret: In most cases, the secret to shaping up and scoring the results you've always wanted boils down to sweating smarter, not harder.

FOCUS ON FORM

If you've been going to the gym regularly and not seeing great results, it may be because you're unknowingly mangling your moves (no offense). Experts agree that proper form is the single most important factor in injury prevention, yet many women don't give it a lot of thought—especially when they're in a rush.

The truth is, most people make tiny but key errors in their techniques, and these mistakes prevent them from building muscle and burning more calories. And it starts with even the most basic, fundamental exercises. That's why if you walked into many of the most elite gyms in the country you'd find trainers putting their clients through staples like these four—over and over until they master the movements. Here's where most people get tripped up and what to do differently.

LUNGES

The main mistake most people make is leaning forward, causing the front heel to rise. To avoid this, start by narrowing your starting stance. The closer your feet are, the harder your core has to work to stabilize your body. Then, as you do the lunge, focus on moving your torso only up and down, not pushing it forward. (It can help to think about dropping your back knee straight down to the floor.) This keeps your weight balanced evenly through your front foot, allowing you to press into the floor with your heel, which tones more lower-body muscles.

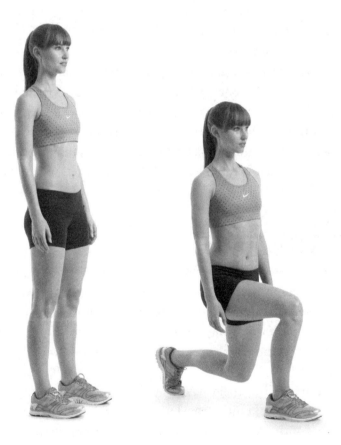

SQUATS

A lot of people's first thought is "bend your knees," when it should be "sit back." Women tend to lean forward on their toes instead of sitting back into their heels. Try this fix: Pretend that you're standing on a paper towel and imagine trying to rip the towel apart by pressing your feet onto the floor and outward. This activates your glutes, which helps you break through plateaus. As you squat, imagine you're sitting down into a chair, rather than forward on top of your knees. Push your hips back first instead of beginning by bending your knees, which puts more stress on your joints. Then, as you stand, think about pushing the floor away from your body, rather than lifting your body.

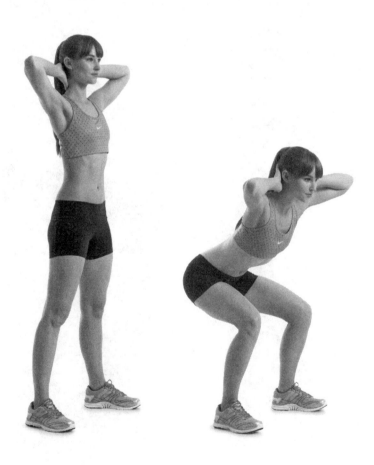

STRAIGHT-LEG DEADLIFTS

It's easy to put too much space between the weight and your body as you move up and down. Pretend you're shaving your legs with the bar or dumbbells. The farther the weights are from your body, the more strain on your back, which limits the work of your hamstrings and glutes. When bending down, act as if you are holding a tray of drinks and need to close the door behind you with your backside. This helps you push your hips back instead of rounding your lower back—a form blunder that puts you at risk for back problems. As you return to standing, squeeze your glutes. You'll engage your butt rather than strain your lower back.

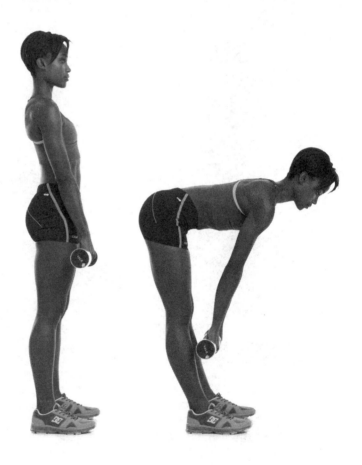

BENT-OVER ROWS

The top mistake here is ignoring the muscles that draw back your shoulder blades. Before you start the exercise, create as much space as you can between your ears and shoulders. Pull your shoulder blades down and back, which will ensure that you work the intended middle- and upper-back muscles. Imagine that there is an orange between your shoulder blades. As you pull the weights or your body up, "squeeze the juice out of it" by bringing your shoulder blades together, and stick out your chest, which allows you to better retract your shoulder blades, which will lead to better results.

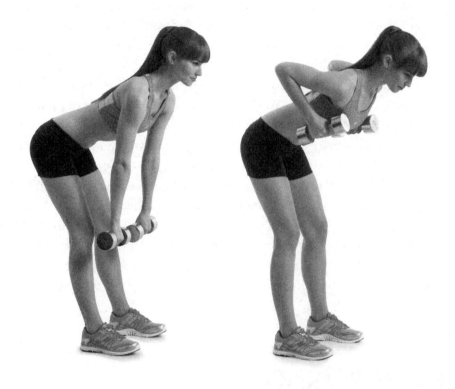

LIFT HEAVY

Dumbbells, resistance bands, even water—they're all ways to apply external force to your workout to make any routine more challenging. The added stress encourages muscle growth, which helps increase your metabolism and blast fat. But in order to get a tighter, leaner body, the chosen resistance has to actually tax your muscles.

This means saying goodbye to feather-light dumbbells. I'm not saying that lifting lighter weights is completely ineffective. Researchers found that lifting 30 percent of your all-out max can be as effective as 80 percent of your max but, and here's the important part, only as long as you complete enough reps to tire out your muscles. Translation: It's going to take considerably more reps at a lighter weight to match the effectiveness of heavier weights. But, again, it comes back to your goal. If it is faster fat loss, supersizing your dumbbells is a better use of your gym time. Hoisting heavier weights builds lean muscle in less time, plus research shows that you can burn nearly twice as many calories in the 2 hours after lifting heavier weights.

And don't even think about skipping the last few reps—this is where the magic happens, so to speak. You have to stress your muscles if you want them to change, and that occurs during those last few reps of the exercise. (If you don't have access to a gym with a range of weights, you want to at least try to have two sets available for any total-body session because your large muscle groups (think legs, glutes, chest, and back) can handle a much larger amount of weight than smaller muscle groups (like your arms, shoulders, and calves) can. Your last reps of any exercise should be tough to finish, but not so difficult that you have to compromise your form. If you're well under the rep range, decrease the weight by 2 to 5 pounds. And if you're busting out 15 to 20 reps with no trouble at all, it's time to increase the challenge by—yep, you guessed it—adding more weight.

USE MORE MUSCLE

Many women, especially if they're new to strength training, stick to a handful of the same exercises (things like biceps curls, calf raises, and crunches). They eventually work a good amount of muscles, head to toe, but it takes a while because they're using what's known as isolation exercises, which only focus on one muscle group at a time.

When you listen to some of the top sports performance coaches in the country—Mike Robertson, Eric Cressey, and Mike Boyle are just a few names that come to mind—their opinions have a familiar theme: Even if the end goal is simply to look great in a bikini, women would benefit from a more athletic training approach. The strength work of athletes places a significant emphasis on movements that we replicate in real life—like squatting, pushing, stepping, jumping, and pulling—rather than just body parts or single muscle groups. Also referred to as "functional training," these big-body exercises help you move bigger weights and build more muscle. At the same time, this movement-centered approach improves mobility, meaning your muscles and joints are able to withstand the stress placed on them during workouts and throughout each day without getting injured.

But you won't just move better and feel stronger: Exercises targeting multiple muscle groups at once (called compound exercises) recruit more muscle fibers, which translates to a higher calorie burn in less time. This functional

STOP PLAYING FAVORITES

Here's one gym shortcut you never want to take: selective strength training. The ever-popular philosophy known as "spot reducing" is a shortcut dieter's dream: It states that if you exercise a specific muscle group, you'll burn fat in that area. Don't love your thighs? Just keep lunging and they'll get leaner. Trying to lose your belly? Bang out enough crunches and the fat will melt right off.

Sound too good to be true? That's because it is. Fat and muscle are two completely independent tissues. Training every day by doing endless crunches and planks will strengthen those muscles, but it won't directly impact the fat surrounding them to flatten your belly faster. To reveal a tight, flat stomach, you need to build more lean muscle all over, which

increases your metabolic rate (the number of calories you burn daily) and helps you shed stubborn body fat faster.

But there's also a subtler variation of spot reduction—something I like to call wish-list workouts. Instead of zeroing in on a single muscle group, they choose exercises that target a few areas—like, say, triceps, abs, and thighs. On the surface, this looks (and probably feels) like a total-body workout. And yes, it increases your body's fat-burning potential because you're engaging a higher percentage of muscle fibers compared to training only one muscle. But working out this way might neglect some crucial supporting players and create muscular imbalances, which can have a big impact on your results.

GET MORE FROM YOUR BODYWEIGHT

Continually fit people know that even when you don't have equipment, you can still get in a great workout. The best know how to tailor bodyweight exercises to their own fitness level—and then adapt them when that level changes. Steal their science-backed rules to get more effective workouts sans equipment.

RULE #1: TO GET LEANER, BE LONGER

As you increase the distance between the point of force (your target muscles) and the end of the object you're trying to lift (your body), you decrease your mechanical advantage. Translation: The longer your body, the weaker you become and the more your muscles have to work. This is the major difference between "girly" pushups and regular ones. When you do pushups on your toes, your core muscles have to work a whole lot harder to support more of your body weight.

APPLY IT / Raise your hands above your head so your arms are straight and in line with your body during lunges, squats, crunches, and situps. Too hard? Split the distance by putting your hands behind your head.

RULE #2: TAKE THE SPRING OUT OF YOUR STEP

When you lower your body during any exercise, your muscles build up what's known as elastic energy. It works like a coiled spring: The elasticity allows you to bounce back to the starting position and reduces the amount of work your muscles have to do.

APPLY IT / Take a 4-second pause at the bottom position of any exercise. That's how long it takes to discharge all the elastic energy of a muscle. Without the bounce, you'll force your body to recruit more muscle fibers to get you moving again.

approach also makes your body a stronger, more efficient unit, so you can challenge it more (read: work it harder and see results faster). Take a look at your workout; no less than 50 percent of the exercises should be big-body moves, as opposed to isolated (or single-joint) exercises.

DITCH THE MACHINES

Free weights, such as barbells and dumbbells, challenge your body more than machines do, according to a study in the *Journal of Strength and Conditioning*

RULE #3: GO THE DISTANCE

Physics defines work as force (here, that's how much you weigh) times distance. Since you can't increase force beyond your own body weight without an external load (like a dumbbell), the only way to work more is to move farther during each rep.

APPLY IT / For bodyweight exercises—such as lunges, pushups, and situps—your range of motion ends at the floor. The solution: Move the floor farther away. Try placing your front or back foot on a step when doing lunges, or position your hands or feet on a step when doing pushups.

RULE #4: ADD A TWIST

Human movement happens on three geometric planes: the sagittal plane (front-back and up-down), the frontal plane (side to side), and the transverse plane (rotation). Many common bodyweight exercises—such as squats and side lunges—are performed on the first two planes. But we rarely train our bodies on the transverse plane, despite using it all the time in our everyday lives, such as when we walk.

APPLY IT / Simply rotate your torso to the right or left during exercises such as lunges, situps, and pushups; you'll fully engage your core in addition to the muscles those moves are intended to target.

RULE #5: GET OFF THE FLOOR

The less of an object's surface area (in this case, your body) that touches a solid base (the floor), the less stable that object is. Fortunately, we have a built-in stabilization system: our muscles. So knocking yourself a little off kilter makes you exercise harder and enlists more muscles.

APPLY IT / Hold one foot in the air during pushups, squats, and planks.

Research. They engage more muscles, increase your range of motion, and are less likely to cause injury. Still, many women spend the majority of their time at the gym hopping from one exercise machine to the next. Next time you hit the gym, sub in these replacement exercises, instead.

SEATED LEG EXTENSION MACHINE

Sure, you'll strengthen your quads—but at a cost. The resistance is close to your ankle, which puts a high amount of torque on your knee when you raise and lower the weight. The result? Kneecap pain. Try a split squat, instead. This move puts less stress on your knees, plus it works your hamstrings and glutes.

Step one foot 3 to 4 feet in front of the other (A), then bend your knees and lower your back knee toward the floor (B). Press through the heel of the front foot to stand. Do 10 reps, then switch legs and repeat.

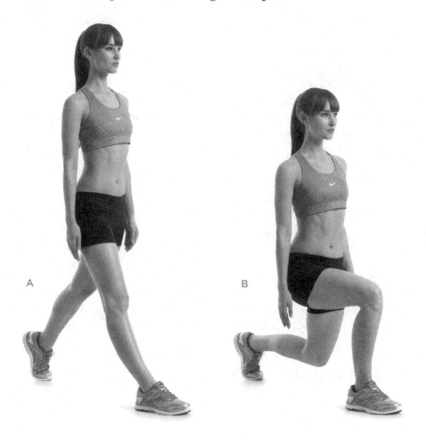

A

B

SEATED ABS CRUNCH MACHINE

Simply put, spinal flexion (the act of bending forward as you do during a crunch) is the cause of most adult back pain. Think of it like a credit card: Bend the card once and it probably won't break. But bend it 100 times and see what happens. And, by adding weight, this machine places even more pressure on your spinal discs, increasing the risk of pain and injury. Instead, do a stability-ball rollout. Your core is meant to stabilize your spine, not move it, and this exercise engages your entire core to keep your spine neutral. Kneel on the ground and place your forearms on a stability ball, palms together (A). Brace your core and slowly roll the ball away from you, keeping your back flat (B). Slowly pull the ball back to the starting position. That's 1 rep. Work up to 20.

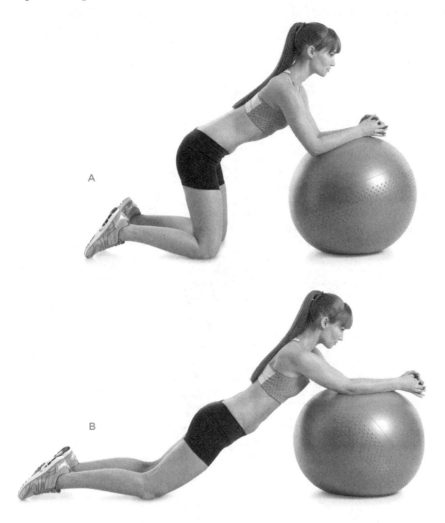

HIP ADDUCTOR/ABDUCTOR MACHINE

Sitting down and squeezing your legs together or pushing them apart won't shrink your thighs no matter how many reps you bang out. These are nonfunctional, unnatural movement patterns that really offer zero payoff. And the abductor move could irritate your iliotibial band, the ropey piece of connective tissue that runs from the outside of your hip to the outside of your knee. A better option: the lateral band walk. Lateral band walks tone the outer thighs, glutes, and hips. Place a small resistance loop above your ankles and sidestep to the right for 15 feet. Step to the left to return to the starting position. That's 1 set. Repeat 2 more times.

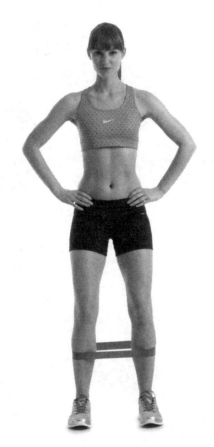

BICEPS CURL MACHINE

The biggest problem here is that it's so easy to cheat! People often rely on gravity to lower (read: drop) from the bar, and cutting your range of motion short not only makes the exercise less effective, but it also causes muscle tightness and strains your elbows and wrists. Replace it with the band-assisted chin-up.

This move hits your biceps, back, shoulders, and core and strengthens the muscles that help you stand tall, so you look longer and leaner. Loop a resistance band around a chin-up bar, threading one end through the other and pulling it tight. Grab the bar with a shoulder-width, underhand grip, place your knee in the loop of the band, and hang at arm's length (A). Pull yourself up to the bar (B). Work up to 10 reps.

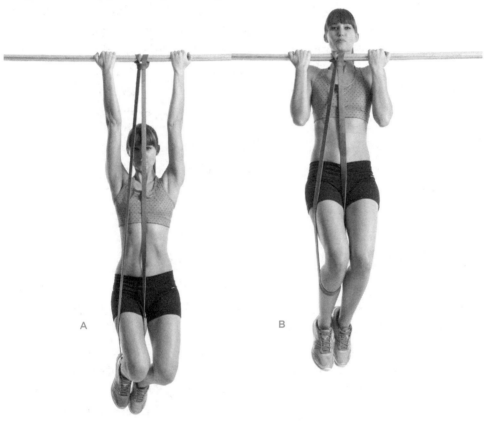

POWER UP

Muscle strength isn't the only thing that can jump-start a sluggish metabolism. Muscle power (sometimes referred to as speed-strength by trainers) is about generating as much force as fast as possible, and it can be a useful weight-loss tool.

In fact, doing a workout that incorporates explosive movements, commonly referred to as plyometrics, is one of the most effective ways to torch calories and burn serious fat. Plyometrics also fire up your fitness level by improving your coordination and agility. They can even boost your speed: Researchers at the University of Nebraska found that participants who improved their vertical jump also logged significantly faster 10K running times.

Whether they're jumps or quick upper-body movements, plyometric exercises increase the elastic properties of your muscles, which, over time, allows them to handle intense workloads more efficiently. The result: Your muscles adapt to more challenging workouts faster, so you see body-shaping results sooner.

Because these types of exercises can be higher impact and harder on your joints, ease into them slowly; when starting a new plyo routine, do it only once a week for the first 2 weeks.

PICK UP THE PACE

When you hit the gas pedal during your workouts—sprinting as fast as you can or doing as many reps as you possibly can—your body becomes less efficient and has to burn more calories to do the activity. Obviously, it's much harder to maintain that all-out effort for an extended period of time, which is why the best fat-fighting strategy is one that involves short bursts of activity that require you to breathe so hard you can't utter a word, followed by easier moves that let you catch your breath.

These quick-but-killer efforts—what have now been collectively referred to as high-intensity interval training (or HIIT, for short)—may be the closest thing you'll find to a magic calorie-burning bullet. Not only do you spend less time working out (which is kinder to your body), but you also continue to incinerate calories at an increased rate during the recovery periods. This kind of training also builds muscle, prevents plateaus, and increases endurance. And that's just the physical payoff: It also busts boredom, boosts confidence, and improves mental toughness, giving you the strength to keep going when your body wants to stop.

WATCH YOUR SPEED

If you think pace only matters when you're out on a run, think again: The speed of your resistance training matters, too. But it may be one of the most overlooked building blocks to an effective strength-training routine.

In the weight room, tempo training refers to the speed at which you lift and lower resistance during an exercise, and adjusting that speed is a great way to get more out of every rep. Sometimes this means moving through exercises more quickly: Researchers at Anderson University and Ball State University in Indiana found that exercisers who performed a weightlifting workout at a quick, explosive pace expended 70 more calories, on average, than those who did the workout at a normal pace.

But you can also score benefits from slowing down your workouts. Your muscle has three main types of contractions: eccentric (lengthening of muscle fibers during the lowering portion of an exercise, like lowering into a squat), isometric (muscle length staying the same while under tension, like the bottom position of a squat), and concentric (the shortening of muscle fibers during the lifting portion of the exercise, like standing up from a squat). Slowing down during the eccentric portion of an exercise can help improve body awareness and stability, as well as stimulate the muscle fibers differently by placing them under more stress. The *Journal of Strength and Conditioning Research* found that an eccentric tempo (taking 3 seconds) significantly increased the amount of calories that both trained and untrained individuals burned for up to 72 hours post-workout. The slow eccentric phase increases the tension on the muscle, which creates a higher calorie

STAY STRONG LONGER

Research shows that plyometrics may also be the key to stronger bones. Your bones constantly go through a rebuilding process to maintain a healthy density. And the best way to trigger that rebuilding is by stressing them with explosive movements, according to a review in *Sports Medicine.* Bone density peaks between ages 25 and 30 and then decreases by 1 to 2 percent a year, so the higher your bone density is before it begins thinning, the lower your risk for osteoporosis later on.

As valuable as high-intensity work-outs are, a little goes a long way—and you don't want to OD on them. Adding extra speed more than once a week can increase your risk for injuries. Slip just one of these pace-pushing workout strategies into your weekly routine. And don't just stick with the one that feels easiest—it's best to mix and match various methods to keep your body guessing.

burn during and after exercise in order to repair the muscles.

And, yes, you can even burn calories without moving a muscle. It's called isometric training, after that second muscle contraction where the muscle length stays the same while under tension. Take a wall squat, for example: Your quads are constantly under stress, even though they don't move. This can be an especially useful strategy for people who lack stability or are dealing with injuries.

Like other pieces of your workout program, you should mix up tempos so your body doesn't adapt to the pace.

REST LESS

If you walk into any weight room, you'll likely find a handful of people standing around not doing much that resembles working out. I can still remember spending up to an hour at a time in my high school weight room over the summer to prepare for field hockey preseason. I used to think that made me sound impressive, but I probably spent 70 percent of the time sitting around "resting" between sets and watching all the football players do the same. It was tedious and slow, and it certainly didn't feel like the most effective workout.

Way back then, I overlooked a crucial point: Just because my legs needed a break after squats didn't mean my whole body did. With the right program, you can take advantage of that downtime by training another muscle group. Take supersets: two exercises that work opposing muscle groups, performed back to back without rest (for example, a chest press combined with a bent-over row). Supersets accomplish more work in a shorter period of time without compromising the effort of each set. In fact, a study in the *Journal of*

Strength and Conditioning Research found that participants burned 33 percent more calories after doing supersets compared with sets that let you rest between moves.

Another popular method: circuit training. This is when you move through a series of strength exercises, going from one to the next with little to no rest. It's a simple shortcut that cuts your gym time in half without cutting corners on your results. What's more, minimizing your downtime between moves also keeps your heart rate elevated and helps maximize the fat-burning impact of your workout. And you know what's more impressive than spending an hour in the weight room? Spending only 30 minutes—and getting an even better workout.

STEADY AT ANY SPEED

Regardless of what tempo you're moving at, one thing should stay the same: You never want to train at a speed that compromises control. When any workout cranks up the intensity or speed, quality can take a back seat to quantity. People sometimes get too focused on banging out as many reps as they can, however they can—even if it means sacrificing form. While the occasional slam of a weight stack is par for the course when using resistance equipment like the cable machine, lowering the weight without control can result in injury. It can also prevent you from getting the results you're after, because you don't work through your full range of motion. With every exercise, make sure your primary objective is proper form—then you can worry about tempo.

TEAM UP

Whether you're looking to tackle your first half-marathon or shape up before your summer vacation, there's one crucial step you can't afford to skip: Building a support network. In fact, after setting the goal itself, this may be the most important factor for success. Research shows that having people in your corner makes you more motivated, more engaged, and—ultimately—more successful. They help motivate you, push you, and keep you accountable. They can offer perspective when you hit bumps in the road, and they can pull you through when you don't think you can keep going. Training with a partner can simultaneously motivate and distract you during tough workouts, which can help you score better results. A study from the University of Pittsburgh reports that women who joined a weight-loss program with a pal lost one-third more

PUSH YOUR LIMITS

When it comes to short-and-sweet workouts, your comfort may need to take a back seat.

Researchers at McMaster University found that exercising as hard as you can for short periods of time is just as effective at improving muscle and metabolism as sweating it out longer at a lower intensity. The Tabata method, for example, involves fast-and-furious intervals—20 seconds of all-out effort followed by 10 seconds of rest—repeated a total of eight times. That's a whopping 4 minutes.

The problem is, without someone egging you on, you may hit the brakes as soon as your workout gets the slightest bit uncomfortable (unlike the study participants, who were killing it during 30-second intervals). When it comes to high-intensity effort, you have to force your body past the point of wanting to quit—a point trainers call volitional fatigue, or when you can't do another rep with perfect form.

Keep in mind, though, that your brain will want to quit before your muscles do: Researchers have found that before you even start working out, your brain is figuring out how to pace your body so that you stop exercising long before you have an issue. Translation: You probably always have more in the tank than your brain leads you to believe.

While the world's most hard-driving athletes know how to ignore that fake-out and get more from their bodies, most of us can't help but fixate on our achy legs and burning lungs. But if that's all you think about, your brain can produce a stress response that increases the ache. So give yourself a mental pep talk before you hit the gym. Remind yourself of how strong and capable you are. If that doesn't work, try one of these research-backed tricks: Mentally repeat the word *smooth* with each pedal stroke on a bike or continuously count up to eight during a run (known as rhythmic cognitive behavior); sing a favorite song or go over your grocery list (distraction or dissociation); or remind yourself that this sprint or strength-training interval will be over in just 30 more seconds (establishing an end).

weight than those who went solo. But there's a subtle—and crucial—aspect to the approach that's often overlooked: Not just any workout buddy will do; it has to be one who will push you. That doesn't mean it always has to be someone right by your side, either: In a 6-month study, dieters who used Twitter to read and post updates and encouraging messages were more likely to succeed than nontweeters.

KEEP TRACK

Research has found that the more people log their weight and exercise, the more weight they lose (and the less they regain—if any). Review your previous workout before you hit the gym and try to find one way to do better. This doesn't mean shaving minutes from your personal record every time you run a 5K. It's as simple as adding an extra rep, going up 5 pounds in the weight room, or running or biking just a little bit longer (another minute or two) after you think you absolutely can't. Progress, no matter how small, is what will get your body changing. Keeping a log also allows you to see how far you've come and keeps you motivated to continue pushing. It's like your personal pat on the shoulder.

QUICK TIPS: TRAINING

40 **Break it up.** Turns out, research has shown the ideal rest time between strength-training sets depends on your goal. For muscle gains, a 2- to 3-minute break is best. To shore up endurance or your metabolic rate, drop it to 60 seconds, max. For best results, include a mix of both methods in your training, say study authors.

41 **Pump up the jams.** People completed an average of 10 additional reps while listening to their favorite music, according to a study from the College of Charleston in South Carolina.

42 **Get your butt in gear.** If your hamstrings cramp up during the glute bridge, it could be a sign that your glutes are weak and your hamstrings are having to work extra hard to keep your hips raised off the ground. Hold each rep for 3 to 5 seconds.

43 **Get off the floor.** Standing upper-body exercises activate your core, tone multiple muscle groups, and increase functional strength, which helps with everything from opening a heavy door to swinging a tennis racket, according to one study.

44 **Strengthen your glutes.** Researchers have found that, in people with knee pain, butt muscles didn't fire properly while running or walking up and down stairs, which may place greater stress on the knees.

45 **Don't forget hip extensions.** Hip extensions hit 55 percent more of your hamstring muscles and 79 percent more of your glute muscles than squats, according to a study by the American Council on Exercise.

46 **Focus on the whole.** People lost twice as much fat when they trained their entire body 3 days a week, compared to working each muscle group only once a week, according to University of Alabama scientists.

47 **Maximize your muscle groups.** You can save even more time during supersets by pairing noncompeting muscle groups (think upper and lower body). So while your arms take a break from biceps curls, your legs can get busy doing squats—which means fewer, and even shorter, rest breaks.

48 **Keep your heels down.** You can point your toes outward up to 30 degrees if it helps you keep your heels on the floor while lifting.

49 **Stay slow and steady.** A new study shows that low-impact martial arts may offer an afterburn effect similar to the one caused by lifting weights. Compared with brisk walkers, people who did tai chi for 45 minutes five times a week saw a greater bump in resting energy expenditure. Researchers say the slow, controlled moves can improve muscle tone and boost metabolism— while also reducing stress, which is linked to fat storage and unbalanced food choices.

ONLY YOU CAN STOP YOU.

FITNESS FIX

PART II

DO THE
WORK

6/

Five-Minute Quick Fix

HERE'S THE THING ABOUT the relationship between time and exercise: Even if everyone could find 5 free minutes each day (and I'll safely assume most can), the majority of us wouldn't use that time to work out.

Why not? For starters, most women assume that 5 minutes isn't enough time to achieve anything significant. (Which, I should point out, I'm not altogether arguing with.) Then, there's the fact that not many workout programs are created for super-short time frames. So what ends up happening is, the ambitious few with a something-is-better-than-nothing attitude do a few minutes of crunches, pushups, and lunges in their living room while they watch TV. Better than nothing? Sure, I guess. Best they can do? Not even close.

The workouts in this chapter are designed specifically for those days when you're short on time—or unmotivated, or tired, or can't make it to the gym. Five exercises, 5 minutes. That's all it takes to rev up your metabolism and build lean muscle.

Just like sprints on a treadmill or in spin class, you have to push hard and fast the entire time. That's what helps dial up the calorie burn and leaves a lingering impression on your metabolism. But while plenty of exercises can leave your lungs burning and muscles aching in the same amount of time, these moves are designed based on an intentional selection of movement patterns that, when paired together, give you an effective and balanced total-body workout. (I like to call them POM-style workouts, which stands for "purpose of movement.") In as little as 5 minutes, these workouts will help you build functional, balanced strength—and, of course, kick-start your fat burners.

Intentionally minimal—you won't need anything more than dumbbells (one heavier and one lighter, if possible) and a bench or step—these workouts are adaptable to your needs. They can be used as solid filler workouts to help maintain consistency when your schedule is hectic. And when you're not pressed for time, they make great back-pocket workouts for when you get to the gym with no plan and need something effective and easy to remember. You can just repeat the same workout three to five times for a full-length circuit workout. Or mix and match a few of the workouts for a longer session that has a wider variety of moves.

MAXIMIZE EVERY MINUTE

Pick one of these two intervals to complete any of the following workouts. Both burn calories, build muscle, and blast fat, but each generates a slightly different metabolic response. Switching between them not only helps speed up results, but it also offers just enough variety to fight mental fatigue.

30:30

Complete as many reps as you can in 30 seconds, then rest for 30 seconds before moving on to the next exercise. (Rest for 60 seconds at the end if you're doing more than one round.) Choose the heaviest weights that will allow you to work for the entire time and maintain proper form but still challenge you to complete the set.

50:10

Complete as many reps as you can in 50 seconds, then rest for 10 seconds before moving on to the next exercise. (Rest for 60 seconds at the end if you're doing more than one round.) You'll need to use lighter weights, but because you'll be able to perform more reps, it should still be tough to finish a set.

QUICK FIX 1

1 STEP UP WITH KNEE DRIVE (LEFT) /

Stand in front of a step or bench and place your left foot on top of it (A). Push down through your left heel, pressing your body straight up onto the bench while driving your right knee up (B). Reverse the movement to return to the starting position. That's 1 rep.

2 STEP UP WITH KNEE DRIVE (RIGHT) /

Repeat this above exercise using the opposite leg.

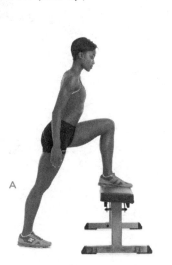
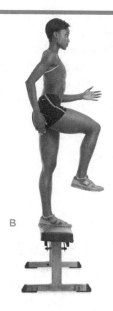

A

B

3 ALTERNATING BENT-OVER ROW /

Hold a pair of dumbbells and stand with your feet hip-width apart. Bend forward at your hips to lower your torso toward the floor, letting the dumbbells hang at arm's length directly from your shoulders (A). Without raising or rotating your torso, pull the right dumbbell toward your chest (B); pause, then lower your right arm (that's 1 rep) while rowing the left weight toward your chest. Continue alternating.

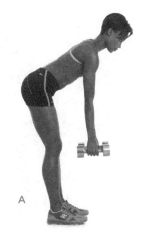
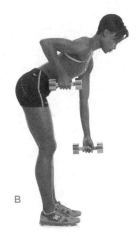

A

B

4 PUSHUP / Place your hands shoulder-width apart on the floor and extend your legs behind you so your body forms a straight line from head to heels (A). Lower your body until your chest nearly touches the floor (B). Pause, then push back to the starting position as quickly as possible. That's 1 rep.

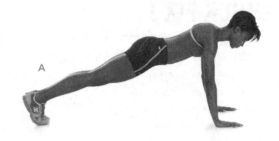

A

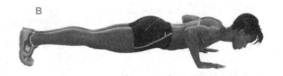

B

5 DUMBBELL SQUAT AND OVERHEAD PRESS /
Hold a pair of dumbbells at shoulder height and stand with your feet hip-width apart, then sit your hips back and lower into a squat (A). Push through your heels to stand, pressing the dumbbells overhead (B). Lower the weights to the starting position. That's 1 rep.

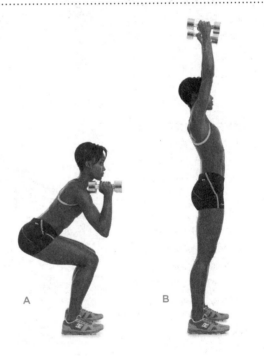

A   B

QUICK FIX 2

1 MARCHING GLUTE BRIDGE /

Lie on your back with your knees bent, feet flat on the floor. Rest your arms on the floor, palms up. Raise your hips so your body forms a straight line from shoulders to knees (A). Brace your abs and lift your right knee toward your chest (B). Hold for 2 seconds, then lower your right foot. Repeat with the other leg. That's 1 rep.

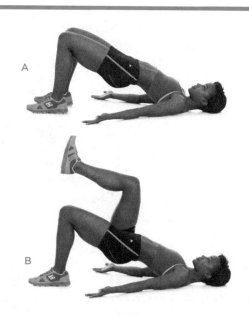

2 INVERTED SHOULDER

PRESS / Start in a pushup position, hands slightly wider than shoulder width, then move your feet forward and raise your hips so your body forms an upside-down V (A). From that position, bend your elbows to lower your body until your head nearly touches the floor (B). Pause, then push back to the starting position. That's 1 rep.

» *Place your feet on a step or bench to increase the challenge.*

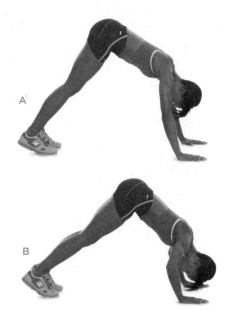

3 ALTERNATING SWITCH
LUNGE / Step your right leg forward and bend both knees to lower into a lunge (A). Press through your right heel to return to standing, keeping your foot lifted, then immediately step your right foot back and lower into a lunge (B). Press through your left heel to return to standing. That's 1 rep.

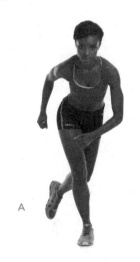
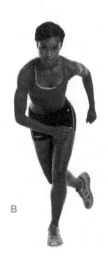

A
B

4 SKATER HOPS /
Stand on your left foot with your left knee slightly bent and your right foot slightly off the floor (A). Jump to the right and land on your right foot, bringing your left foot off the ground (B). That's 1 rep. Jump to the left and continue alternating as quickly as possible.

A
B

5 ROTATING T EXTENSION /

Start in a pushup position (A). (Make it harder by adding a pushup here.) Keeping your arms straight and your core engaged, shift your weight onto your left arm, rotate your torso to the right, and raise your right arm toward the ceiling so that your body forms a T (B). Hold for 3 seconds, then return to the starting position and repeat on the other side. That's 1 rep.

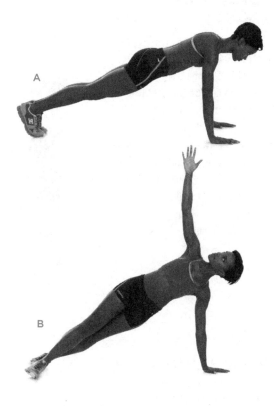

A

B

QUICK FIX 3

1 DUMBBELL SPLIT JERK /

Hold a pair of dumbbells at shoulder height, palms facing each other, feet hip-width apart (A). Dip your knees, then quickly press the dumbbells directly overhead as you jump your legs apart so that you land in a staggered stance, one foot in front of the other (B). Step or jump back to the starting position, lowering the weights back to your shoulders. That's 1 rep.

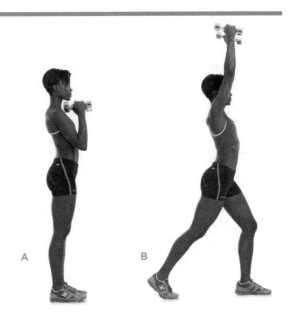

A

B

2 PUSHUP-POSITION ROW /

Get into a pushup position with your hands resting on dumbbells, feet slightly more than hip-width apart (A). Shift your weight back slightly onto the balls of your feet before you start, then pull one weight toward the side of your chest, keeping your hips parallel to the floor (B). Lower and repeat on the other side. That's 1 rep.

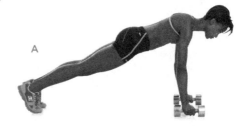

A

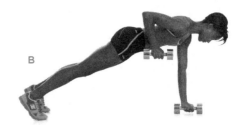

B

3 ALTERNATING LATERAL

LUNGE / Holding a pair of dumbbells at your sides (A), step to the right and bend your right knee to lower into a side lunge, keeping your back flat and lowering the weights toward your right foot (B). Press through your right heel to return to the starting position. That's 1 rep. Repeat on the other side and continue alternating.

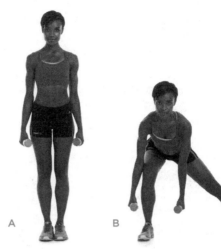

A   B

4 REVERSE WOODCHOP

(LEFT) / Holding a dumbbell with both hands, stand with your feet wider than hip width, bend your knees, and lower the weight to the outside of your left thigh (A). In one motion, press through your heels to stand, and raise the weight over your right shoulder, arms straight and core tight (B). Reverse the movement to return to the starting position. That's 1 rep.

5 REVERSE WOODCHOP

(RIGHT) / Repeat the above exercise, this time starting with the weight to the outside of your right thigh and raising it over your left shoulder.

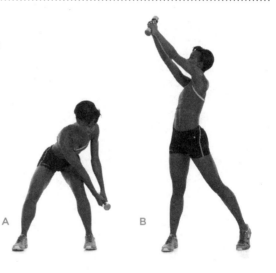

A   B

QUICK FIX 4

1 STRAIGHT-LEG DUMBBELL DEADLIFT / Hold a pair of dumbbells in front of your thighs, feet hip-width apart (A). Push your hips back and hinge forward to lower your torso until it's almost parallel to the floor, keeping the weights close to your body (B). Squeeze your glutes and push your hips forward to return to standing, still keeping the weights close to your body (as if you're shaving your legs with the dumbbells). That's 1 rep.

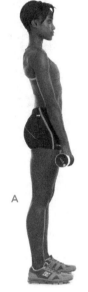

A

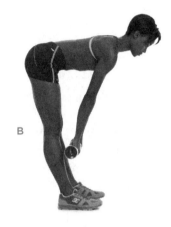

B

2 OVERHEAD DUMBBELL SPLIT SQUAT (RIGHT LEG) /

Grab a pair of dumbbells and stand with a step or bench about 2 feet behind you. Bend your left knee to place the top of your foot on the step or bench and raise the weights overhead, arms straight and core tight (A). Bend your knees to lower your body toward the ground (B). Push through your right heel to stand. That's 1 rep.

Your hips should stay directly under your body throughout this exercise. Think "drop down" not "lunge forward."

3 OVERHEAD DUMBBELL SPLIT SQUAT (LEFT LEG) /

Repeat the above exercise, starting with your right foot on the bench.

» *Holding the weights overhead increases the demand on your core. If your form starts to falter at any time, bend your elbows to bring the weights to shoulder height, or lower your arms to your sides and continue.*

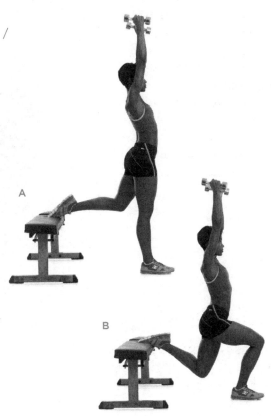

A

B

4 SIDE-TO-SIDE JUMPS /

Stand with your arms at your sides, feet together and knees slightly bent (A). Jump to the left with both feet together (imagine you're jumping over a 5-inch cone) (B), landing softly on the balls of your feet; that's 1 rep. Immediately jump to the right, and continue going back and forth as quickly as possible.

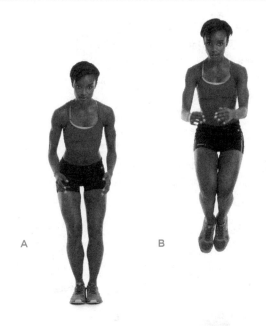

A

B

5 CROSS-BODY MOUNTAIN CLIMBER /

Start in a pushup position, core and glutes engaged (A). Keeping your back flat and hips level, bend your right knee toward your left shoulder (B). Return to the starting position and repeat with your left leg. That's 1 rep.

A

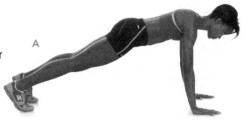

B

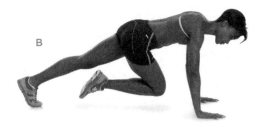

QUICK FIX 5

1 BENT-KNEE DEADLIFT /

Set a pair of dumbbells on the floor in front of you. Keeping your chest lifted, sit back and bend your knees to squat down and grab the dumbbells with an overhand grip (A). Press through your heels, squeezing your glutes and pushing your hips forward to stand (B). Slowly reverse the movement to lower the dumbbells to the floor. That's 1 rep.

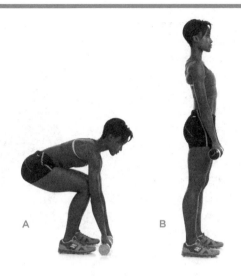

A   B

2 SINGLE-ARM ROTATIONAL ROW (RIGHT ARM) /

Stand with your left foot about 2 feet in front of your right, holding a dumbbell in your right hand, palm facing your body. Bend your knees and hinge forward to lower your torso toward the floor, the weight hanging straight from your shoulder (A). Brace your core and pull the dumbbell toward the right side of your chest, rotating your torso to the right (B). Pause, then lower back to the starting position. That's 1 rep.

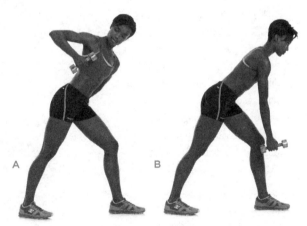

A   B

3 SINGLE-ARM ROTATIONAL ROW (LEFT ARM) / Repeat the
above exercise, this time with the weight in your left hand and your right foot in front of your left.

4 GOBLET SQUAT WITH ROTATION AND PRESS /

Stand with your feet slightly wider than hip width and hold a dumbbell vertically in front of your chest, with both hands cupping the dumbbell head (A). Bend your knees and push your hips back to lower your body until your thighs are parallel to the ground. In one motion, stand up and rotate your feet and torso to the left as you press the weight over your left shoulder (B). Reverse the movement to return to the starting position and repeat to the other side. That's 1 rep. Continue alternating.

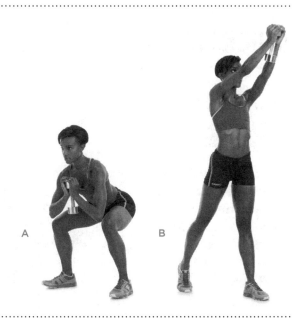

5 PLANK DUMBBELL DRAG /

Place a dumbbell on the floor and get into a pushup position, feet slightly wider than hip width, weight outside your left hand (A). Keeping your core tight and hips parallel to the floor, reach your right hand under your body, grab the weight, and pull it to the right (B). Place your right hand back on the floor (C). That's 1 rep. Reach your left arm under your body and repeat on the other side; continue alternating.

>> *The weight of the dumbbell increases the difficulty of this move. If you're unable to maintain proper form (keeping your hips parallel to the floor and your body in a straight line), use a lighter dumbbell. You can also complete this as a bodyweight exercise (simply reaching underneath your body to the other side) to build core stability before adding a dumbbell.*

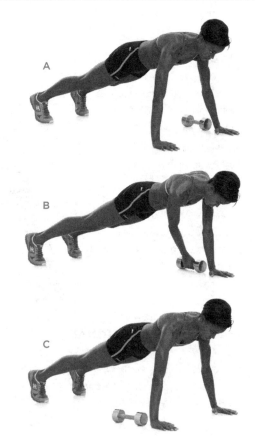

QUICK FIX 6

1 SUMO SQUAT WITH LATERAL RAISE /

Grab a pair of dumbbells and stand with your feet wider than shoulder-width apart, toes turned out. Sit your hips back and bend your knees to lower into a squat, arms straight and dumbbells between your knees, palms facing each other (A). In one motion, press through your heels to stand and raise both dumbbells to shoulder height (B). Slowly reverse the movement and immediately lower into another rep.

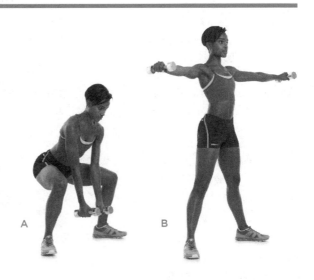

2 DUMBBELL CHEST PRESS /

Grab a pair of dumbbells and position your upper back on a bench with your knees bent and feet flat on the floor. Raise your hips to form a straight line from shoulders to knees, and press the dumbbells over your chest, arms straight and palms facing away from you (A). Lower the weights until your upper arms are in line with your chest (B). Press back to the starting position. That's 1 rep.

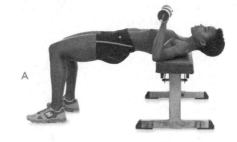

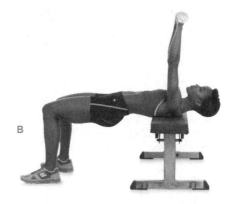

» This variation recruits more of your glutes, hamstrings, and core throughout the exercise. You can make it easier by lying completely on the bench; you can make it harder by swapping the bench for a stability ball. But don't forget the goal of this exercise: to challenge your chest and arms. So choose a variation that allows you to lift a challenging weight with proper form.

3 PLANK WALKUP /

Position your forearms on the ground, elbows directly under your shoulders, and extend your legs behind you (A). Keeping your back flat and hips parallel to the floor, place your right hand flat on the floor (B), and then your left hand, straightening your arms to press your body into a pushup position (C). Reverse the movement, lowering onto your right forearm and then your left, to return to the starting position. That's 1 rep. Repeat, leading with your left hand, and continue alternating.

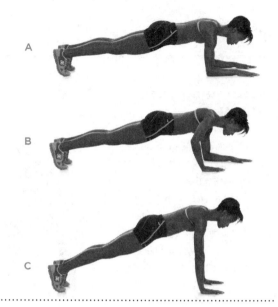

4 DUMBBELL LUNGE WITH ROTATION /

Grab a dumbbell with both hands and raise it to shoulder height in front of you, arms straight and feet hip-width apart (A). Keeping your core tight and your chest up, step forward with your left foot and lower your body until your front thigh is nearly parallel to the floor, rotating your shoulders and torso to the right (B). Rotate back to the center as you press through your right heel to return to the standing position. That's 1 rep. Repeat on the other side and continue alternating.

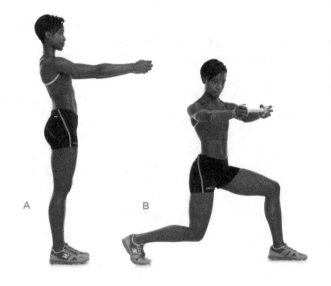

» If at any point during the interval it's too difficult to keep your arms straight out in front of you, bring the weight close to your chest and continue as directed. Still too challenging? Ditch the dumbbell and complete the remaining reps as a bodyweight move.

5 LOW-BOX LATERAL
SHUFFLE / Stand to the right of a low box or step and place your left foot on it; bend your knees slightly and keep your chest up (A). Push off your left foot and jump over the box to your left, landing with your right foot on the box and your left foot on the floor, knees bent (B). Quickly return to the starting position. That's 1 rep.

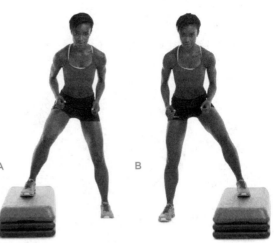

A

B

QUICK FIX 7

1 WEIGHTED GLUTE BRIDGE /

Lie faceup on the floor with your knees bent and heels on the floor; place a dumbbell across your body, just below your hip bones, and hold it with one hand (A). Tighten your core, contract your glutes and hamstrings, and raise your hips until your body forms a straight line from shoulders to knees (B). Lower to return to the starting position. That's 1 rep.

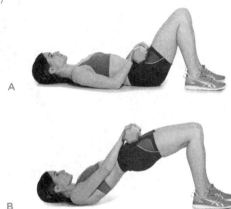

A

B

2 CHEST PRESS WITH FEET ELEVATED /

Lie faceup with hips and knees bent 90 degrees. Hold a pair of dumbbells above your chest, arms straight, palms facing away from you (A). Lower the dumbbells until your upper arms touch the floor (B). Press back to the starting position. That's 1 rep.

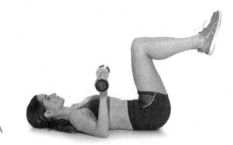

A

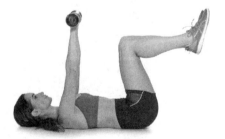

B

3 DUMBBELL FRONT SQUAT /

Stand with your feet shoulder-width apart. Hold a pair of dumbbells so that your palms are facing each other, and rest one end of the dumbbell on each shoulder (A). Keep your body as upright as you can at all times, and keep your upper arms parallel to the floor. Brace your abs and lower your body as far as you can by pushing your hips back and bending your knees (B). Pause, then push yourself back to the starting position. That's 1 rep.

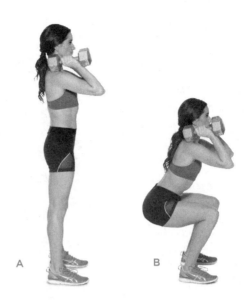

A   B

4 REAR LATERAL RAISE /

Grab a pair of dumbbells and bend forward at your hips until your torso is nearly parallel to the floor. Let the dumbbells hang straight down from your shoulders, palms facing each other (A). Without moving your torso, raise your arms straight out to the sides until they're in line with your body (B). Pause, then slowly return to the starting position. That's 1 rep.

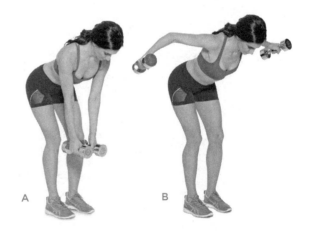

A   B

5 SQUAT JACK / Stand with your feet hip-width apart, hands together and in front of your chest. Bend your knees and sit your hips back to lower your body until your knees are bent nearly 90 degrees (A). From that position, jump your legs out to the side (B); immediately jump back to the starting position. That's 1 rep. Continue, while holding the lowered squat position.

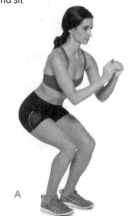

A

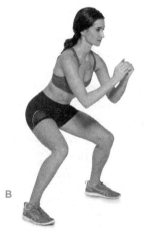

B

QUICK FIX 8

1 HIP THRUST / Sit in front of a bench, knees bent and feet flat on the floor, upper back leaning against the edge of the bench (A). Raise your hips to form a straight line from your knees to your shoulders, with your upper back resting on the bench (B). Pause, then return to the starting position. That's 1 rep.

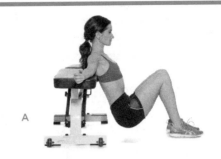

A

B

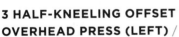

2 HALF-KNEELING OFFSET OVERHEAD PRESS (RIGHT) /
Begin in a half-kneeling position, your left foot flat on the floor in front of you, your right hand holding a dumbbell at shoulder level (A). Keeping your core tight and chest tall, press the dumbbell directly overhead (B). Reverse to return to the starting position. That's 1 rep.

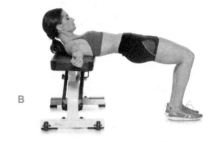

A

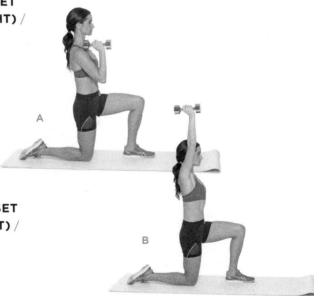

B

3 HALF-KNEELING OFFSET OVERHEAD PRESS (LEFT) /
Repeat the above exercise, this time starting with your right foot flat on the floor in front of you and a dumbbell in your left hand.

4 NARROW-STANCE
BOX SQUAT / Stand about a foot in front of a bench or box, hands at your sides and feet about 6 inches apart (A). Sit your hips back and bend your knees to lower into a squat until your body is fully sitting on the bench (B). Press through your heels to return to standing. That's 1 rep.

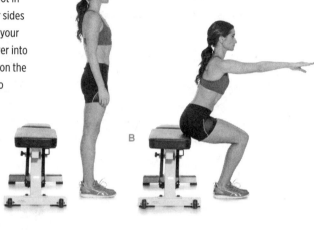

A

B

5 ALTERNATING LATERAL
STEP-UP / Stand to the left of a bench, hands on hips. Cross your left leg in front of your right to place your left foot on the bench, knee bent at 90 degrees (A). Push through your left heel to extend your leg and raise your body to stand on the bench (B). Step your right foot down to the right, then your left; repeat on the opposite side, and continue alternating.

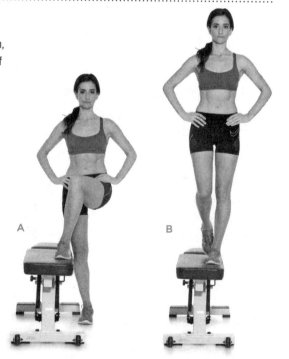

A

B

QUICK FIX 9

1 ALTERNATING REVERSE LUNGE TO OVERHEAD

PRESS / Hold a pair of dumbbells at shoulder height, palms facing in, feet about hip-width apart (A). Step your left foot back and lower your body until both knees are bent to 90 degrees, simultaneously pressing the right dumbbell straight above your shoulder until your arm is straight (B). Reverse the movement to return to the starting position. That's 1 rep. Repeat on the other side, then continue alternating.

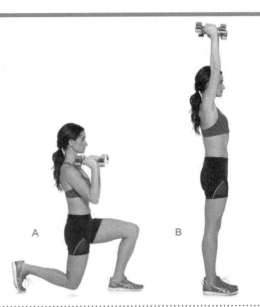

A   B

2 HOT POTATO SQUAT /

Hold a dumbbell in your right hand at shoulder height, elbow bent, and stand with your feet shoulder-width apart. Keeping your chest upright and core tight, sit your hips back and bend your knees to lower into a squat (A). As you press through your heels to stand, gently toss the weight up and over in front of you (B), catching it with your left hand and immediately lowering into another squat. Continue alternating back and forth.

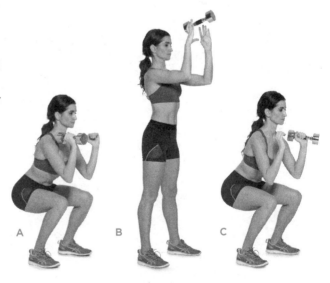

A   B   C

3 ALTERNATING CURTSY

LUNGE / Stand with your feet hip-width apart, hands on hips (A). Keep your chest and eyes up and shoulders squared. Cross your right leg behind your left and bend both knees, lowering your body until your left thigh is nearly parallel to the floor (B). Return to the starting position, then repeat on the other side. That's 1 rep.

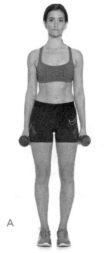
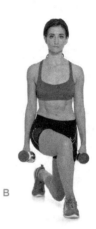

A   B

4 SQUAT POP-UP /

Start in a pushup position, hands under your shoulders and legs extended, body forming a straight line from head to heels (A). Brace your core and jump your feet outside your hands, then quickly lift your chest and hands so that you're upright (B). Reverse the movement to return to the starting position. That's 1 rep.

A
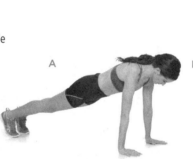
B
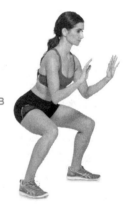

5 DUMBBELL FAST FEET /

Hold a heavy dumbbell with both hands in front of your chest, elbows bent and at your sides. Keeping your core tight, chest tall, and knees softly bent, alternate picking up one foot at a time as quickly as you can, pushing through the balls of your feet.

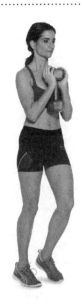

QUICK FIX 10

1 SUMO DUMBBELL

DEADLIFT / Set a pair of dumbbells on the floor in front of you, and place your feet about 3 feet apart, toes turned out. Squat down, keeping your chest up, and grab the dumbbells with an overhand grip. Your arms should be straight and your lower back slightly arched, not rounded (A). Contract your glutes and stand up, lifting the dumbbells, straightening your legs, thrusting your hips forward, and pulling your torso back and up (B). Slowly lower the weights back to the floor. That's 1 rep.

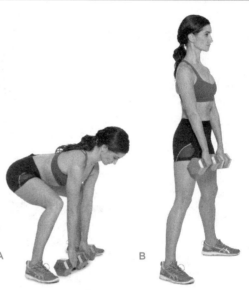

A   B

2 DUMBBELL PUSH PRESS /

Stand tall with your feet shoulder-width apart, holding a dumbbell in each hand at shoulder height, palms facing each other (A). Bend your knees slightly, then explosively push up with your legs as you press the dumbbells over your head (B). Lower the weights to return to the starting position.

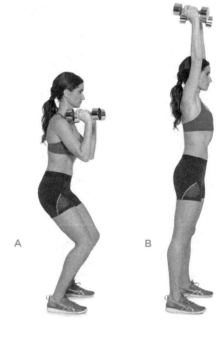

A   B

3 SUITCASE SQUAT /

Hold a pair of dumbbells at your sides, palms facing in (like you're holding two suitcases), and stand with your feet shoulder-width apart (A). Sit your hips back and bend your knees to lower your body until your thighs are nearly parallel to the floor (B). Press through your heels to return to the starting position. That's 1 rep.

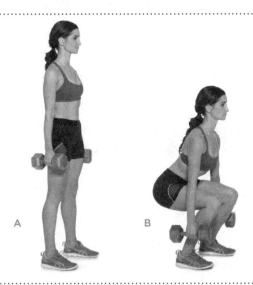

A   B

4 DUMBBELL UNDERHAND

ROW / Grab a pair of dumbbells and stand with your feet shoulder-width apart, knees slightly bent. Bend forward from your hips until your back is almost parallel to the floor, with your arms hanging directly from your shoulders and palms facing away from your body (A). Brace your core, then pull the weights toward your chest, squeezing your shoulder blades together (B). Pause, then lower back to the starting position. That's 1 rep.

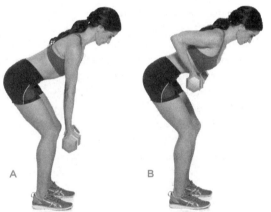

A   B

5 PLANK JACK /

Get into a pushup position, feet hip-width apart and hands about shoulder-width apart (A). Keeping your core tight, jump both feet a few inches farther apart (B), pause, and then jump your feet back together to return to the starting position. That's 1 rep.

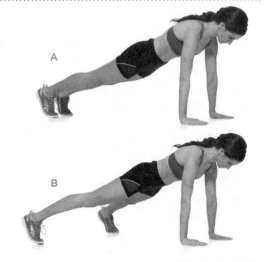

A

B

QUICK TIPS:
RESULTS

50 **Picture it.** Visualizing yourself kicking ass preworkout or race can enhance your performance—but only if you do it right before you start. In a study published in the *Journal of Strength and Conditioning Research,* runners who imagined themselves sprinting superfast up to 2 minutes before a race ran significantly faster than those who didn't. But the effect disappeared if they did the visualization more than 3 minutes before hitting the track. Researchers suspect that having more time between dreaming and doing causes you to lose the psychological momentum you've built. Try it: 30 seconds before your next sweat session, close your eyes and mentally watch yourself rock it.

51 **Rethink your cardio.** Doing cardio before resistance training zaps strength and energy levels fast, so save it for the end of your routine. And if you're running out of time, don't worry about the clock—just go harder. You'll improve your conditioning more by running at a higher intensity for 15 minutes than with a slow, 30-minute jog.

52 **Aim higher.** To help combat the inaccurate calorie-burn counts on some cardio machines, increase your calorie-burn goal by 30 percent. So if you go to the gym with the intention of burning 300 calories, aim for 390, instead.

53 **Roll out before a workout.** Run a rolling massager over your hamstrings before a workout to boost flexibility. Start with two sets of 10 seconds and work your way up to three sets of 20 seconds or more.

54 **Set your playlist in advance.** One survey found that gym-goers spent 30 percent of their workout time doing things like finding the right music and chatting.

55 **Smile like you mean it.** Even a half-hearted grin actually makes demanding situations much more manageable, according to researchers. Plus, you'll look that much better in those photos they snap during the race.

56 Buddy up. In one study, participants who were told their peers held a plank for a second longer than their first one went on to hold their own second try 5 percent longer. Get a boost from your friends by asking them to tell you when they're going to the gym (knowing they're going can get you there, too—which is often the hardest part), or share stats with a few of your friends after your workout.

57 Get fit while you sleep. Take in 20 grams of protein (about 7 ounces of Greek yogurt, for example) after your workout and again 30 minutes before bed to give your body access to much-needed amino acids that can be used to build muscle while you sleep.

58 Get 150 minutes for better sleep. Study participants who completed 150 minutes of moderate exercise (about 30 minutes a day, 5 days a week) fell asleep faster and felt less tired during the day.

STAY POSITIVE. WORK HARD. MAKE IT HAPPEN.

FITNESS FIX

7 / Get It Done in One

IT SOUNDS CRAZY: That you could get an effective workout with just one exercise? But it's true. My colleague—former *Men's Health* fitness director BJ Gaddour—has popularized what he calls EMOM (or "Every Minute on the Minute") workouts. They deliver strength and conditioning—all by using one move and a 1-minute interval.

The approach is simple: Simply choose one exercise and decide how many reps you'll complete each round. (Ten reps works better for slower moves like squats or pushups, and 20 reps works better for faster moves like swings or skater jumps. For really challenging moves like pullups, you can go as low as 5 reps EMOM, while for pure cardio moves—like jumping jacks—you can go as high as 50 to 100 reps per minute.) Then start a timer and complete all your reps in less than 1 minute, resting for any time that's left over. That's one round. The faster you finish your reps, the more time you'll have to rest. When the timer hits 1 minute, repeat; then continue until you've completed all your rounds. (A general guideline: Complete anywhere from 10 to 30 rounds for a 10- to 30-minute workout. Or choose a few exercises and complete in two or three separate 10-minute workouts. Only have a few minutes? Do as many rounds as you have time for!)

It's that easy. And it's plateau proof: You can progress each time by using heavier weights or by increasing your rep-per-minute goal.

While almost any exercise can work, here are 10 of my favorites.

SQUAT PRESS / Stand with feet shoulder-width apart and hold a dumbbell horizontally with both hands close to your chest, keeping your elbows next to your sides (A). Push your hips back and bend your knees to lower your body as far as you can into a squat. From that position, extend your arms straight out in front of you (B), then bring them back to your chest and press through your heels to return to the starting position.

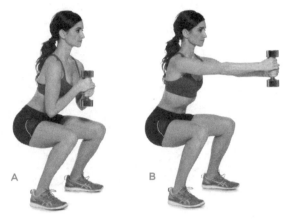

A　　　　　　B

SQUAT TO OVERHEAD PRESS / Stand holding dumbbells at your shoulders, elbows bent, feet hip-width apart, and palms facing each other. Push your hips back and bend your knees to lower your body until your thighs are nearly parallel to the floor (A). As you stand, press the weights overhead until your arms are straight (B). Lower the weights to your shoulders to return to the starting position.

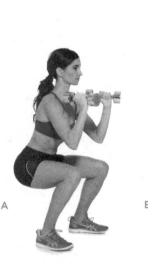
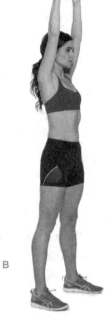

A　　　　　　B

KETTLEBELL SWING /

Stand with your feet shoulder-width apart, a kettlebell on the floor in front of you. Bend your knees, push your hips back, and grab the top of the kettlebell with both hands. Without arching your lower back, swing the weight back between your legs (A). Then squeeze your glutes, thrust your hips forward forcefully, and swing the weight to chest height (B). Let it fall back through your legs to complete 1 rep, then continue swinging, allowing momentum to move the weight rather than your arms.

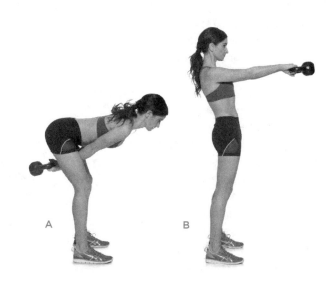

PUSHUP / Start on all fours with your

hands slightly wider than and in line with your shoulders. Lift your knees off the ground and straighten your legs, feet close together, to form one straight line from your head to heels (A). Brace your abs as you bend through your elbows to lower your body until your chest nearly touches the floor, your upper arms forming a 45-degree angle with your body (B). Pause, then push yourself back to the starting position as quickly as possible.

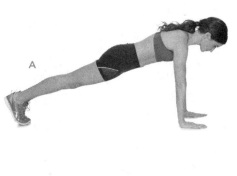

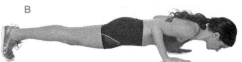

DUMBBELL THRUSTERS /

Stand with your feet shoulder-width apart, and hold a dumbbell in each hand above your shoulders, elbows out and palms facing each other. Push your hips back and bend your knees to lower your body into a squat until the tops of your thighs are nearly parallel to the floor (A). Lower the weights to the floor (B), maintaining your grip, and tighten your core as you jump your legs back into a pushup position (C). Reverse the movement to return to standing.

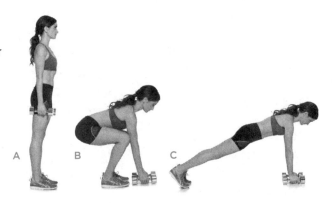

WALKING LUNGES /

Stand tall with your hands behind your head or on your hips (A), then step forward with your right leg and slowly lower your body until your front knee is bent 90 degrees and your back knee almost touches the floor (B). Keeping your torso tall, press through your right heel to bring your left foot forward to return to standing. That's 1 rep. Alternate the leg you step forward with each time.

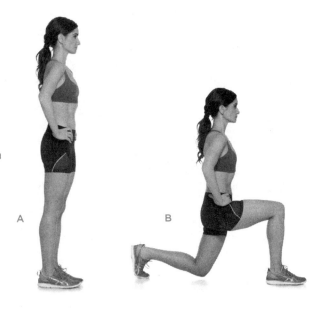

DUMBBELL CLEAN /

Stand with your feet shoulder-width apart and a dumbbell between your feet on the floor. Push your hips back as you squat to grab the dumbbell with your right hand, arm fully extended (A). In one smooth movement, pull the weight up and "catch" it at shoulder height as you press through your heels to stand (B). Pause, then reverse the movement to return to the starting position. Complete all reps, then switch sides and repeat.

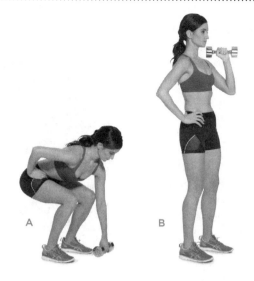

A

B

DUMBBELL PUSH PRESS /

Stand tall with your feet shoulder-width apart, holding a dumbbell in each hand at shoulder height, palms facing each other (A). Bend your knees slightly, then explosively push up with your legs as you press the dumbbells over your head (B). Lower the weights to return to the starting position.

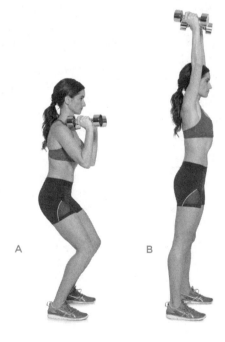

A

B

DUMBBELL PISTON PUSH-PULLS /

Stand with your feet shoulder-width apart, holding a dumbbell vertically with both hands, arms extended. Bend your knees slightly and hinge forward at your hips so that the weight is between your knees. This is the starting position (A). Keeping your back flat and core tight, bend your elbows to pull the weight up toward your body (B); pause, then push the weight away from you until your arms are straight.

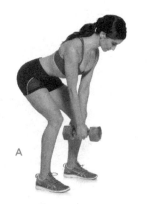

A

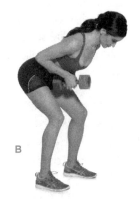

B

SKATER HOPS / Stand on your left foot with your left knee slightly bent and your right foot slightly off the floor. Jump to the right and land on your right foot, bringing your left foot off the ground (A). That's 1 rep. Jump to the left, raising your right foot (B), then continue alternating as quickly as possible.

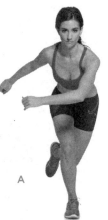

A

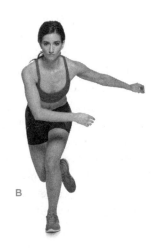

B

QUICK TIPS:
ACTIVE HABITS

59 **Commute car-free.** Commuters racked up an additional 14.6 minutes of physical activity each day that they took public transit, according to a study in the *American Journal of Public Health.* If you can't ditch your car, try to add 15 minutes of exercise by taking walking business calls on your cell, parking further from the grocery store, and using the stairs.

60 **Give a green thumbs-up.** Research has found that 30 minutes of medium-high intensity gardening tasks (think planting, hoeing, and weeding) can satisfy the government's daily exercise recommendations.

61 **Take the stairs.** In one study, when 69 hospital employees used the stairs exclusively for 12 weeks, those steps added up to a 1.7 percent decrease in body fat, a 1.8 percent decrease in waist circumference, a 3.9 percent decrease in LDL cholesterol, and an 8.6 percent increase in lung capacity.

62 **Be a weekend warrior.** Research in the *Journal of Obesity* found that adding 20 minutes of activity on Saturday or Sunday leads to 1.6 percent less body fat over a year. The researchers say we consume more calories on the weekend, which exercise can help offset, and even minor movement usually leads to more.

CELEBRATE THE LITTLE VICTORIES.

FITNESS FIX

8 / Simple Workouts That Work

THERE'S A LOT OF fitness equipment out there. It's all over infomercials, your local gym, maybe even your home. And there are some terrific tools to help make you stronger, faster, and leaner, while creating more dynamic, fun, and effective workouts. With the right combination, you can amplify your body's innate ability to build muscle and burn fat—and see even more impressive results.

But sometimes even with a dream team of equipment, the sum of their individual genius doesn't add up to an unmatched workout. In fact, when you need a stability ball, step, kettlebell, cable machine, and resistance band—all for one 20-minute workout—the time it takes to set up from one piece of equipment to the next can lower the overall intensity—not to mention tack on precious minutes to your total gym time.

The innovative routines in this chapter are created by some of the top trainers in the country, and each is scientifically designed to give you the most effective workout in under 30 minutes—using only one piece of equipment (or none!). It's all about simplicity—dialing back the extras in your sweat session so you can make the most out of every rep, every set, every minute. And without fumbling from one piece of equipment to the next—or worse, waiting to work out during rush hour at the gym—you'll save time with each workout. So whether you're in a crowded gym or at home with basic equipment, there's a routine that will work for you.

BODYWEIGHT

You don't need a gym membership to sculpt a great body. In fact, you don't even need equipment. Think about the classic pullup—for many women, it's freakin' hard to do, and yet there are no weights involved. That's because when you do a pullup, your body is in a position that forces your back and arms to lift your entire bodyweight, so the scientific laws of motion and leverage are working against you. In other words, physics turns your body into an über-efficient resistance machine.

The problem is, just like with any exercise routine, over time your body adapts and basic bodyweight exercises—like squats, pushups, and, yes, even pullups—become easier. Increasing the number of reps can offset the plateau, but only to an extent.

This workout, created by Mark Verstegen, world-renowned athletic performance specialist and founder of Athletes' Performance in Phoenix, has three distinct phases that increase in difficulty so you can keep seeing results. During each phase, you'll move quickly through four compound sets; like their cousin the superset, compound sets are an incredible time-saver because they transition from one move to the next with no downtime. Unlike supersets, which work two opposing muscle groups back to back, compound sets work the same muscle group. Take the first two moves, for example: a bodyweight squat followed immediately by an isometric wall squat. This back-to-back pattern helps recruit even more muscle fibers and creates greater strength gains—all without adding external resistance (think: dumbbells).

Here's how to do it: Start with Workout 1. Refer to the instructions for Phase 1 in the box on the opposite page and complete the prescribed number of reps for A1 and A2, moving from one to the next without rest; move on to B1 and B2 and repeat, and continue until you've finished all of the exercises. A full round of all four compound sets is considered one circuit. Rest for 60 to 90 seconds, then repeat for two to four total circuits.

There are three ways to make this workout more difficult (aka, to keep seeing progress and avoid hitting plateaus): First, you can increase the volume by moving through the three phases using the same workout but increasing the reps and duration. Or you can also increase the exercise difficulty by going from Workout 1 to Workout 2 to Workout 3 but keeping the phase the same. Lastly, you can change both factors—volume and exercise difficulty—at the same time: Start in Phase 1 with Workout 1, then move to Phase 2 with Workout 2, and finally Phase 3 with Workout 3. The choice is yours!

PHASE 1	PHASE 2	PHASE 3
A1 • B1 • C1	A1 • B1 • C1	A1 • B1 • C1
10 REPS	**15 REPS**	**20 REPS**
A2 • B2 • C2 • D1 • D2	A2 • B2 • C2 • D1 • D2	A2 • B2 • C2 • D1 • D2
30 seconds (or 15 each side)	**40 seconds** (or 20 each side)	**60 seconds** (or 30 each side)

WORKOUT 1

A1 BODYWEIGHT SQUAT /

Stand with your feet slightly wider than hip-width apart, and raise your arms straight in front of you at shoulder height (A). Keeping your arms straight and your chest lifted, sit your hips back and bend your knees to lower your body until your thighs are parallel to the ground (B). Pause, then press through your heels to return to standing. That's 1 rep.

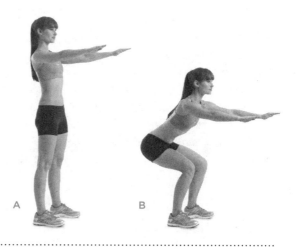

A   B

A2 ISOMETRIC WALL SQUAT /

Stand with your back against a wall, your feet about 2 feet in front of you, hip-width apart. Bend your knees to lower your body until your knees are bent at 90 degrees. Hold.

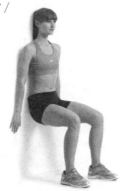

B1 MODIFIED WIDE-GRIP
PUSHUP / Start in a pushup position
with your hands wider than shoulder-
width apart on the floor, then place your
knees on the ground, so your body forms
a straight line from shoulders to knees (A).
Bend your elbows to lower your body
toward the floor in a straight line (B).
Press back up to the starting position.
That's 1 rep.

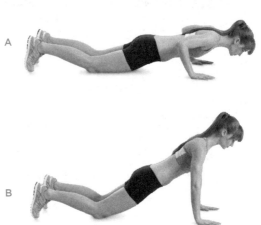

A

B

B2 NARROW-GRIP
MODIFIED ISOMETRIC
PUSHUP / Start in a pushup position
with your hands closer than shoulder-width
apart on the floor, then place your knees on
the ground, so your body forms a straight
line from shoulders to knees. Bend your
elbows to lower your body until your
elbows form 90-degree angles. Hold.
(Keep your shoulders safe by imagining
that you're trying to push the ceiling up
with your back, without moving your arms.)

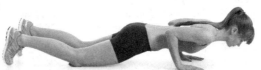

C1 SPLIT SQUAT / Stand with your legs staggered, your right foot about 2 feet in front of your left (A). Bend your knees to lower your body until your right thigh is parallel and your shin is perpendicular to the floor (B). Straighten your legs to return to the starting position. That's 1 rep. Complete all reps on that leg, then switch sides and repeat.

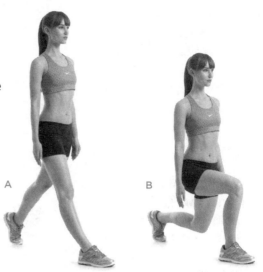

A

B

C2 GLUTE BRIDGE / Lie faceup on the floor with your knees bent, feet flat on the floor, and arms to your sides, palms facing up. Press through your heels and raise your hips off the ground so your body forms a straight line from shoulders to knees. Hold.

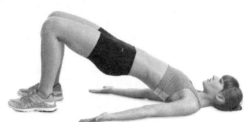

D1 PLANK / Place your forearms on the ground with your elbows directly under your shoulders, and extend your legs so that your body forms a straight line from head to heels. Brace your core and hold.

D2 INCHWORM / Stand with your feet hip-width apart, bend over, and touch the floor in front of your feet with both hands (A). Keeping your legs straight and core tight, walk your hands forward as far as you can without letting your hips drop (B, C). Pause, then slowly walk your feet toward your hands. That's 1 rep.

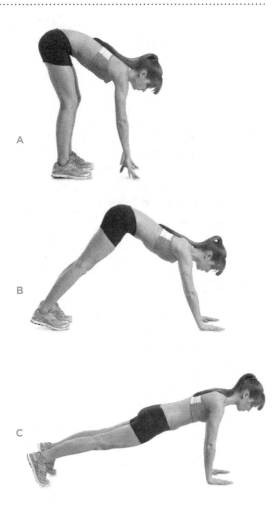

A

B

C

WORKOUT 2

A1 ALTERNATING LATERAL LUNGE / Stand with

your feet hip-width apart, arms raised to shoulder height (A). Keeping your arms raised and your chest lifted, step out to the right with your right leg; bend your knee and sit back to lower into a side lunge, keeping your back flat (B). Press through your right heel to return to starting position. That's 1 rep; repeat on the other side and continue alternating.

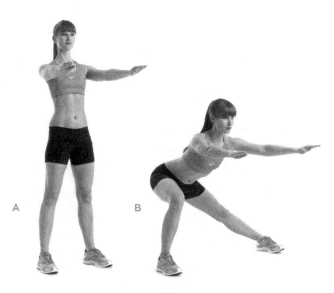

A   B

A2 ALTERNATING SINGLE-LEG ISOMETRIC WALL

SQUAT / Stand with your back against a wall, your feet about 2 feet in front of you, hip-width apart. Bend your knees to lower your body until your knees are bent at 90 degrees (A). Extend your right leg out in front of you, shin parallel to the floor (B). Hold for 1 or 2 seconds, then switch sides and repeat. Continue alternating.

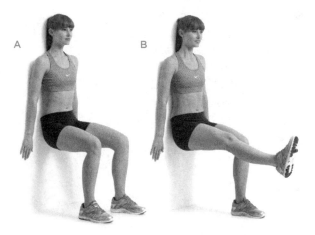

A   B

B1 WIDE-GRIP PUSHUP /

Place your hands on the floor wider than shoulder-width apart, and extend your feet behind you into a pushup position, so your body forms a straight line from head to heels (A). Bend your elbows to lower your body toward the floor in a straight line (B). Press back up to the starting position. That's 1 rep.

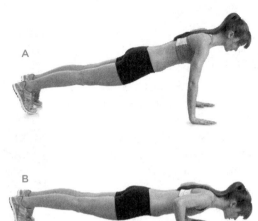

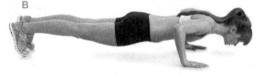

B2 NARROW-GRIP ISOMETRIC PUSHUP /

Place your hands on the floor closer than shoulder-width apart, and extend your feet behind you into a pushup position, so your body forms a straight line from head to heels. Keeping your core tight, bend your elbows to lower your body in a straight line until your elbows form 90-degree angles. Hold.

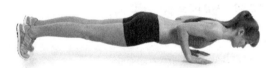

C1 REVERSE LUNGE /

Stand with your feet hip-width apart, arms at your sides (A). Step back with your left leg and lower your body until your right knee is bent at 90 degrees (B). Push back up to the starting position. That's 1 rep. Complete all reps on that leg, then switch sides and repeat.

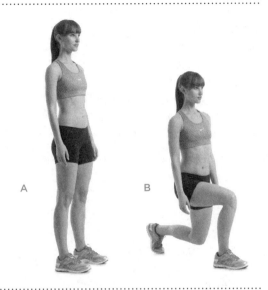

A

B

C2 MARCHING GLUTE BRIDGE /

Lie faceup on the floor with your knees bent, feet flat on the floor, and arms to your sides, palms facing up. Press through your heels and raise your hips off the ground so your body forms a straight line from shoulders to knees (A). From this position, raise your right foot off the ground, knee bent at 90 degrees, until your shin is parallel to the floor (B). Hold for 2 or 3 seconds, then lower your right foot and repeat with the left foot. Continue alternating.

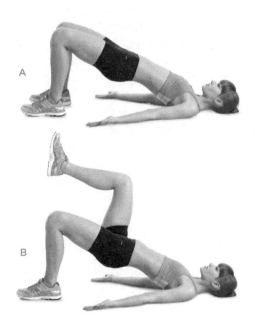

A

B

D1 SIDE PLANK / Lie on your left side and place your forearm on the ground with your elbow directly under your shoulder, your legs straight, and both feet on the floor. Lift your hips so your body forms a straight line from head to heels. Hold, then switch sides and repeat.

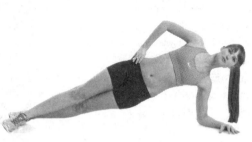

D2 INCHWORM WITH PUSHUP / Stand with your feet hip-width apart, bend over, and touch the floor in front of your feet with both hands (A). Keeping your legs straight and core tight, walk your hands forward until they are directly under your shoulders and your body forms a straight line from head to heels (B). Bend your elbows to lower your chest to the ground (C), then straighten your arms; slowly walk your feet toward your hands. That's 1 rep.

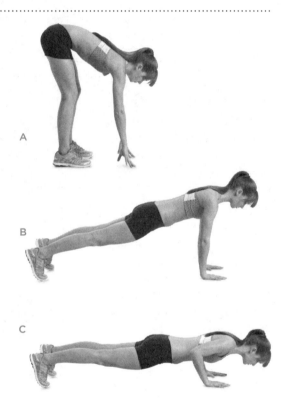

A

B

C

WORKOUT 3

A1 SINGLE-LEG BODYWEIGHT SQUAT /

Stand with your feet hip-width apart, arms raised to shoulder height (A), and raise your left foot off the ground. Keeping your arms raised and your chest lifted, sit your hips back and bend your right knee to lower your body as far as you can, keeping your left leg extended off the ground in front of you (B). Press through your heel to return to standing. That's 1 rep. Complete all reps on that leg, then switch sides and repeat.

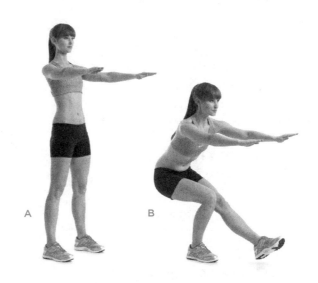

A   B

A2 SINGLE-LEG ISOMETRIC WALL SQUAT /

Stand with your back against a wall, your feet hip-width apart about 2 feet away from the wall. Bend your knees to lower your body until your knees are bent at 90 degrees. Extend your right leg out in front of you, shin parallel to the floor. Hold for 1 or 2 seconds, then switch sides and repeat. Continue alternating.

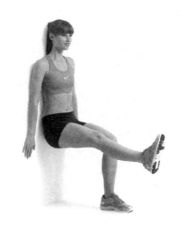

B1 ALTERNATING SINGLE-LEG WIDE-GRIP PUSHUP /

Place your hands on the floor wider than shoulder-width apart, and extend your feet behind you into a pushup position, so your body forms a straight line from head to heels. Raise your left leg (A), then bend your elbows to lower your body toward the floor in a straight line (B). Press back up to the starting position and lower your leg. That's 1 rep. Repeat on the other side and continue alternating.

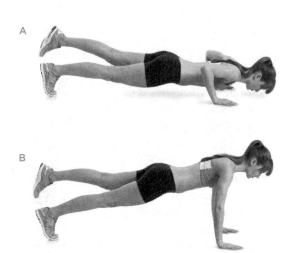

A

B

B2 SINGLE-LEG NARROW-GRIP ISOMETRIC PUSHUP /

Place your hands on the floor closer than shoulder-width apart, and extend your feet behind you into a pushup position so that your body forms a straight line from head to heels. Raise your left leg, then bend your elbows to lower your body in a straight line until your elbows form 90-degree angles. Hold.

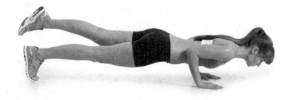

C1 REAR-FOOT ELEVATED
SPLIT SQUAT / Stand about 2 feet in front of a step or bench and place the top of your left foot on it (A). Bend your knees to lower into a lunge until your left knee grazes the floor, keeping your chest upright and hips directly under your body (B). Push through your right heel to stand. That's 1 rep. Complete all reps with that leg, then switch sides and repeat.

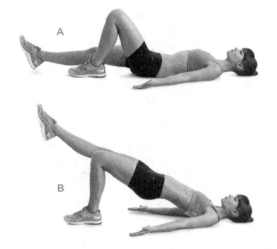

C2 SINGLE-LEG HIP
EXTENSION / Lie faceup on the floor with your left knee bent and your right leg straight (A). Raise your right leg until it's in line with your left thigh. Push your hips upward, keeping your right leg elevated, until your body forms a straight line from shoulders to right ankle (B). Pause, then slowly lower your body and leg back to the starting position. That's 1 rep. Complete all reps with that leg, then switch sides and repeat.

D1 ROLLING PLANK /

Start in the plank position, with your forearms on the ground and your legs extended behind you (A). Rotate your torso to the side, rolling onto your left forearm and into a left-side plank (B). Pause, then return to the starting position, and repeat on the other side.

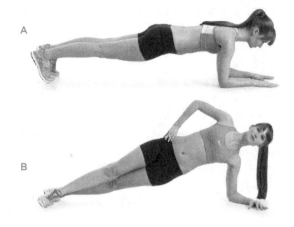

A

B

D2 BURPEE /

Stand with your feet slightly wider than shoulder-width apart, arms at your sides. Push your hips back, bend your knees, lower your body into a squat, and place both hands on the floor in front of you (A). Jump both feet back into a pushup position (B); bring your feet back into a low squat and quickly jump up into the air, swinging your arms overhead and then moving back to standing (C). That's 1 rep.

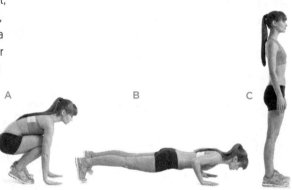

A   B   C

TRX

Looking to shake up your normal routine? Sculpt every muscle in your body with a suspension system like TRX, which creates resistance from two things always at your disposal: body weight and gravity. And it does so at a fraction of the cost of a personal trainer or gym membership.

This portable, affordable tool is a favorite of fitness experts like renowned performance trainer Todd Durkin, CSCS, owner of Fitness Quest 10 and author of *The Impact! Body Plan*. And it's not just reserved for his all-star athletes like Drew Brees; he uses this tool with all of his clients. That's because it's simple yet versatile, allowing Durkin to choose from hundreds of functional exercises to build strength, endurance, core stability, and mobility at any fitness level. (You can simply change the way you position your body to increase or decrease the intensity.) Plus, the suspension trainer forces your core to work harder during every exercise, accelerating your progress toward your flat-belly goals.

Build a stronger, leaner body from head to toe and burn fat fast with this workout created by Durkin. Starting with Circuit 1, complete the prescribed number of reps for each exercise, moving from one to the next without resting. Repeat for a total of three sets, then rest for 2 minutes. Follow the same pattern to complete three sets of Circuit 2, then continue to Circuit 3 and perform two sets.

CIRCUIT 1

TRX SQUAT JUMP /

Grab the TRX handles in both hands and stand facing the anchor point with your arms extended, feet shoulder-width apart (A). Sit your hips back and bend your knees to lower your body until your thighs are parallel to the ground. Keeping your arms straight, press through your heels and quickly jump up as high as you can with both feet off the ground (B). Land softly and immediately lower into another rep. Do 10.

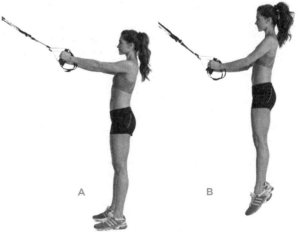

A   B

TRX CHEST PRESS / Stand facing away from the anchor point, feet hip-width apart, and hold the handles in front of you with arms extended at shoulder height, palms facing the floor (A). Walk your feet away from you and lean forward so your body forms a straight line from head to heels. Keeping your core tight, bend your elbows to lower your chest toward the handles (B). Pause, then press back to the starting position. That's 1 rep. Do 10.

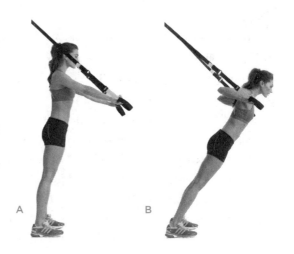

A   B

TRX ROW / Grab the TRX handles in both hands and stand facing the anchor point with feet shoulder-width apart and arms straight in front of you. Lean back and walk your feet forward to the appropriate resistance angle (A). Keeping your shoulders pulled down and back, bend your elbows to pull your chest toward the handles (B). Pause, then return to the starting position with a slow, controlled movement. That's 1 rep. Do 10.

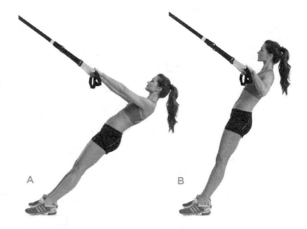

A   B

CIRCUIT 2

TRX BICEPS CURL / Grab the TRX handles in both hands with an underhand grip, and stand facing the anchor point with feet shoulder-width apart and arms straight in front of you. Lean back and walk your feet forward to the appropriate resistance angle (A). Keeping your shoulders down and your body in a straight line, bend your elbows to curl the handles toward your shoulders (B). Pause, then return to the starting position with a slow, controlled movement. That's 1 rep. Do 10.

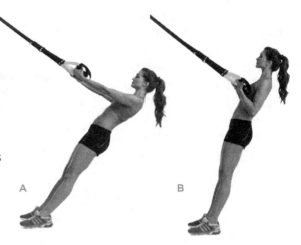

A

B

TRX OVERHEAD TRICEPS EXTENSION / Stand facing away from the anchor point, feet hip-width apart, and hold the handles with your palms facing down and your arms extended (A). Pressing your body weight into the handles, bend your elbows and lower your body until your hands are behind your head (B). Drive your hands forward and extend your arms to return to the starting position. That's 1 rep. Do 10.

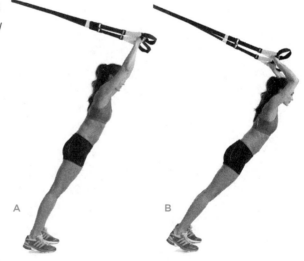

A

B

TRX POWER PULL / Stand facing the anchor point, feet hip-width apart, and hold one handle in your right hand, arm extended at shoulder height. Lean back and walk your feet forward to the appropriate resistance angle (A). Keeping your core tight and your body in a straight line, bend your right elbow to pull your chest toward the handle (B). Pause, then return to the starting position. That's 1 rep. Do 8, then switch sides and repeat.

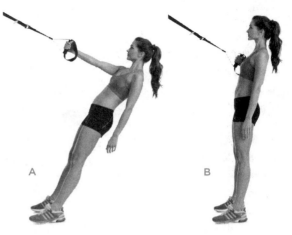

A

B

CIRCUIT 3

BURPEE / Stand with your feet about shoulder-width apart (A), then push your hips back and squat down to place your hands on the floor (B). Jump your legs back into a pushup position (C); quickly reverse the movement to return to the starting position. That's 1 rep. Do 10.

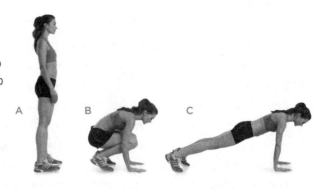

SKATER JUMP / Cross your left leg behind your right and lower into a half-squat, your right arm out to the side, left arm across your hips (A). Hop to the left, switching your legs and arms (B). That's 1 rep. Keep hopping quickly from side to side. Do 30.

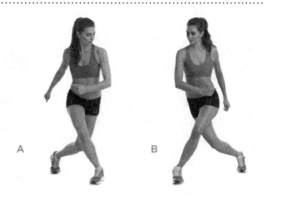

ONE DUMBBELL

This routine—created by Craig Ballantyne, CSCS, a strength and conditioning coach in Toronto and author of *Turbulence Training*—will incinerate fat and tighten your body in record time. Starting with the first exercise, perform the prescribed number of reps, then rest for 30 seconds before continuing to the next move. (You can rest for up to a minute, if needed; make it harder by reducing the rest break or dropping it altogether.) Repeat until you've finished the entire circuit, and rest for 2 minutes. That's one set; aim to finish as many as you can in the time you have, up to 30 minutes. (Beginners should start with two total.)

NARROW-STANCE GOBLET SQUAT /
Stand with your feet shoulder-width apart and hold a dumbbell vertically in front of your chest, both hands cupping the dumbbell head (A). Keeping your chest up and your core tight, sit your hips back and squat as low as you can (B). Press through your heels to return to the starting position. That's 1 rep. Do 15.

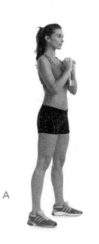
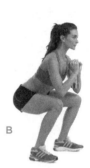

A

B

SINGLE-ARM BENT-OVER ROW /
Place your left knee and left hand on a bench and hold a dumbbell in your right hand at arm's length, palm facing the bench (A). Slowly bend your elbow and pull the dumbbell to your chest (B). Pause, then lower back to the starting position. That's 1 rep. Do 10, then repeat on the other side.

A

B

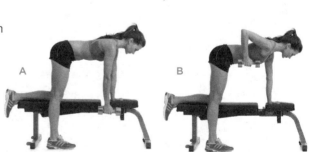

SINGLE-ARM CHEST PRESS /

Lie faceup on a bench, holding a dumbbell in your left hand at chest height (A). Press the weight directly over your shoulder (B). Slowly lower back to the starting position. That's 1 rep. Do 10, then switch arms and repeat.

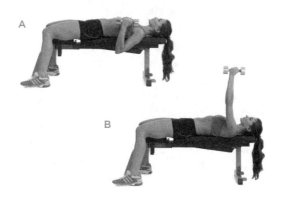

GOBLET SPLIT SQUAT /

Stand with your right foot 2 feet in front of your left and hold a dumbbell vertically in front of your chest (A). Bend your knees to lower your body until your right thigh is parallel to the floor (B). Straighten your legs to return to the starting position. That's 1 rep. Do 6, then switch legs and repeat.

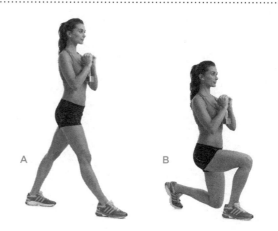

DUMBBELL SWING / Grab a dumbbell with an overhand grip, feet hip-width apart. Push your hips back, knees slightly bent, and lower your chest to bring the dumbbell between your legs (A). Keeping your core tight, push your hips forward and swing the dumbbell up to shoulder height (B). Reverse the movement, swinging the weight back between your legs. That's 1 rep. Do 15.

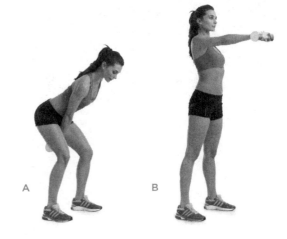

A

B

KETTLEBELL

If you think kettlebells are just hyped-up dumbbells, think again. Unlike a dumbbell, a kettlebell's center of gravity shifts during an exercise, increasing the challenge and building coordination. Researchers found that people who did 20-minute kettlebell workouts torched almost 300 calories—and that's just for starters. When you factor in the calories burned after you exercise, as your body repairs its muscle fibers, the total expenditure could increase by up to 50 percent.

Shed fat fast with this metabolism-boosting kettlebell routine from Tony Gentilcore, CSCS, co-founder of Cressey Performance in Hudson, Massachusetts. Complete the following six exercises in order as instructed, moving from one to the next without rest; rest for up to 60 seconds, and repeat for a total of three to five rounds. Then move to the Finisher: It will take 5 to 10 minutes, but it's the secret to dialing up your metabolism after you're finished.

KETTLEBELL SUMO DEADLIFT / Stand with your feet about twice shoulder-width apart and your toes pointed out slightly. Bend at your hips and knees and grab the kettlebell handle with an overhand grip. Your lower back should be slightly arched, and your arms should be straight (A). Without allowing your lower back to round, pull your torso back and up, thrust your hips forward, and stand up with the kettlebell (B). That's 1 rep. Do 12 to 15.

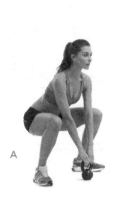

A

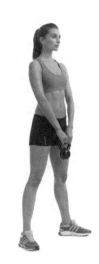

B

KETTLEBELL PUSHUP-POSITION ROW /

Get in a pushup position with your right hand on top of a kettlebell (A). Keeping your hips parallel and back flat, bend your elbow to row the weight toward your chest (B). Pause, then return to the starting position. That's 1 rep. Do 8 to 10, then switch sides and repeat.

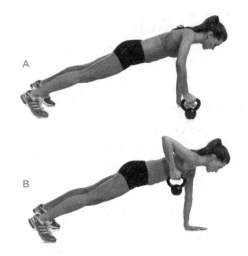

KETTLEBELL REVERSE LUNGE /

Hold the kettlebell handle in your right hand so the bell rests on the back of your forearm (the "racked" position), hand close to your chest and elbow close to your body (A). Brace your core, step back with your right leg, and bend both knees to lower your body until both knees form 90-degree angles (B). Pause, then press through your left heel to return to the starting position. That's 1 rep. Do 10 to 12, then switch sides and repeat.

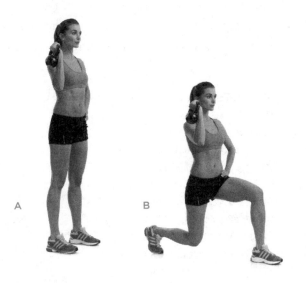

KETTLEBELL HALO /

Stand with your feet hip-width apart and hold the kettlebell in front of your head at about shoulder height (A). Keeping your core tight and stable, circle the weight counter-clockwise around your head (B). Reverse the movement to return to the starting position. That's 1 rep. Do 12 to 15.

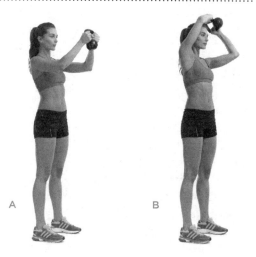

A

B

KETTLEBELL HALF GET-UP /

Lie faceup on the floor with your right knee bent, foot flat on the floor, and your left leg extended straight; hold a kettlebell in your right hand, with your hand directly over your shoulder (A). Roll onto your left forearm and punch the ceiling with your right hand to raise your upper body off the ground (B). Straighten your left arm and place your hand on the floor behind you, so that your upper body forms a T; then press into your right heel and raise your hips until they're in line with your knee, raising the weight toward the ceiling (C). Pause, then slowly reverse the movement to return to the starting position. That's 1 rep. Do 8 to 10, then switch sides and repeat. Don't rush through this exercise. Think of each movement as its own distinct step.

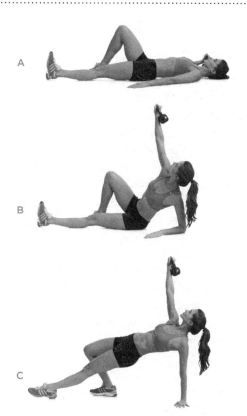

A

B

C

YOGA PUSHUP / Place your hands on the ground directly under your shoulders and extend your legs behind you into a pushup position, with your body forming a straight line from head to heels (A). Bend your elbows to lower your chest toward the ground (B); straighten your arms, and as you return to the starting position, raise your hips up in the air while driving your heels into the ground (downward-facing dog position) (C). Reset to the starting position. That's 1 rep.

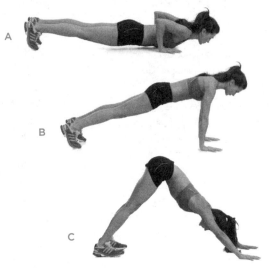

FINISHER »

SINGLE-ARM FARMER'S WALK SHUTTLE WITH KETTLEBELL SWINGS /

Set up two markers roughly 25 to 30 yards apart. Hold a kettlebell at your right side; walk from one marker to the other, keeping your chest upright (A). Once you reach the second marker, position your feet about hip-width apart and hold the kettlebell in front of you with both hands. Push your hips back, slightly bend your knees, and lower your chest to bring the weight between your legs (B). Quickly push your hips forward and swing the weight to chest height (C). Immediately bring the weight between your legs. That's 1 rep. Do 10. Hold the kettlebell in your left hand and walk back to the first marker. Perform another 10 swings. That's one round. Rest for 30 to 60 seconds. Repeat for a total of two to four rounds.

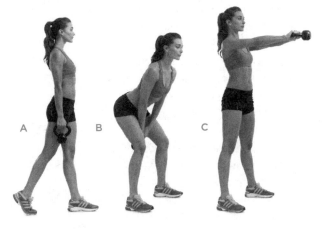

LOW BOX

Crank up your calorie burn and score a fierce physique with this explosive 15-minute workout created by David Jack, director of Teamworks Fitness in Acton, Massachusetts. It takes advantage of a traditional cardio step to strengthen your cardiovascular system and tone your muscles at the same time—the ultimate one-two punch for igniting your fat-burning engine. The innovative dynamic exercises Jack uses help boost agility and speed, and because they aren't likely in your everyday routine, you'll stay more focused on the movements. (You might even have some fun.)

Using a traditional aerobics step (or a 4- to 6-inch low box), perform the following circuit as instructed below. The key is to move quickly while always maintaining proper form; challenge yourself to squeeze out an extra rep each time you complete this routine.

ALTERNATING ELEVATED REVERSE LUNGE / Stand on a step or box (A), then step your left leg onto the floor behind you; bend both knees to lower until your right knee is bent at least 90 degrees (B). Push through your right heel to return to the starting position. That's 1 rep. Repeat on the other leg and continue alternating for 40 seconds. Rest for 20 seconds, then move to the next exercise.

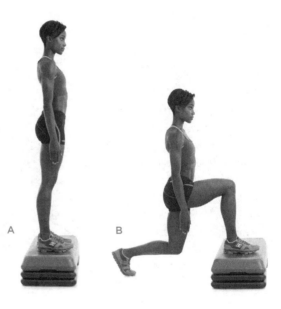

A

B

PUSHUP PLANK WALKOVER /

Start in a pushup position to the right of a low box or step (A). Keeping your body in a straight line from head to heels, place your left hand on the step (B). (Make it harder by adding a pushup.) Then place your right hand on the step (C). Place your left hand on the floor to the left of the step, followed by your right, so that both hands are now on the left side of the step. Reverse to return to the starting position. That's 1 rep. Continue for 10 seconds, then rest for 10 seconds. Repeat three times (1 minute), then move to the next exercise.

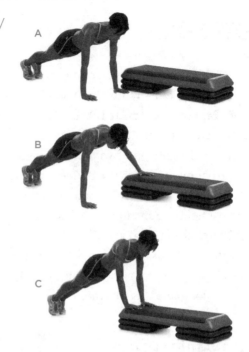

SCISSOR SWITCHES /

Place the ball of your left foot on the step in front of you (A). Press into the box and jump, switching feet so that your right foot is on the step (B). That's 1 rep. Continue alternating as quickly as possible for 10 seconds, then rest for 10 seconds. Repeat three times (1 minute). Rest for 20 seconds, then move to the next exercise.

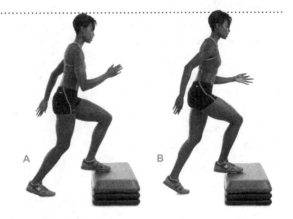

PLANK WITH ALTERNATING LEG RAISE /

Place your forearms on the step, elbows directly under your shoulders, and extend your feet behind you (A). Keeping your core tight and your back flat, raise your right leg off the ground so it's in line with your shoulders (B). Hold for 3 seconds, then lower and repeat with the other leg. Continue alternating for 30 seconds. Rest for 30 seconds, then move to the next exercise.

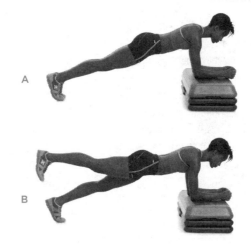

A

B

SQUAT AND POP / Place one foot on either side of the step (the narrow portion between your feet); sit your hips back to lower into a half squat, keeping your chest up (A). Quickly jump both feet up onto the box (B), landing softly and immediately jumping back to the starting position, lowering into another squat. That's 1 rep. Continue for 30 seconds, then immediately move to the next exercise.

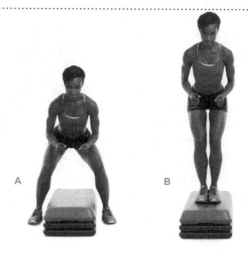

A

B

SIDE PLANK / Place your left forearm on the step directly under your shoulder; extend your legs and raise your hips so that your body forms a straight line from head to heels. Squeeze your glutes and, bracing your core, hold for 20 seconds, then immediately switch sides and repeat. Rest for 20 seconds, then move to the next exercise.

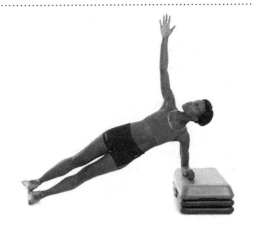

THE RUNAROUND / Stand to the side of the step, knees and elbows slightly bent. Quickly step your left foot onto the step (A), followed by your right, and then quickly step off to the other side, your left foot (B) followed by your right. Reverse the movement to return to the starting position. Repeat the lateral step over, then run forward and make a circle around the entire step. That's 1 rep. Immediately repeat the lateral step overs, and continue this pattern for 40 seconds. Rest for 40 seconds, then repeat the circuit one more time.

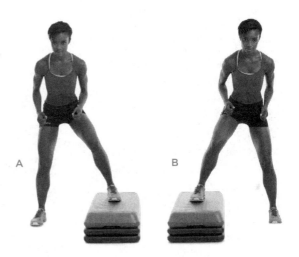

A   B

MEDICINE BALL

Pop quiz: What piece of fitness equipment can you throw, catch, hold, and lift? The correct answer: a medicine ball. (If you answered "a dumbbell," please don't work out near other people.)

Whether you're throwing it onto the ground or catching it midlunge, a medicine ball challenges your core stability and coordination while toning your upper and lower body. This fast-paced circuit workout, created by Hannah Davis, New York City–based personal trainer and co-owner of Gotham Versatile, will blast fat and sculpt muscle in 30 minutes. It's super simple, too: Starting with Circuit 1, complete the prescribed number of reps for each exercise, moving from one to the next without resting. Rest for up to a minute (if needed), then repeat two more times for a total of three circuits. Rest for 1 to 2 minutes, then continue to Circuit 2 and repeat. Continue this pattern until you've finished the entire workout.

CIRCUIT 1

MEDICINE BALL ROLLING PUSHUP / Get into a pushup position with your right hand on top of a medicine ball and your left hand on the floor, your body in a straight line from head to heels (A). Bend your elbows to lower your chest toward the floor (B), then press back up until your arms are fully extended. Roll the ball to your left, then quickly place your weight on your right hand and place your left hand on top of the ball (C). Do another pushup, then roll the ball back to the starting position. That's 1 rep. Do 10 to 14.

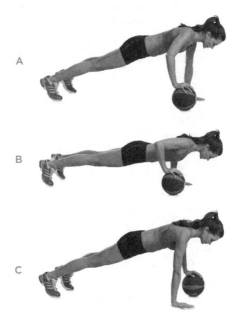

A

B

C

MEDICINE BALL HIP RAISE /

Lie faceup on the floor, arms out to your sides with palms up, and place both feet on a medicine ball, knees bent about 90 degrees (A). Squeeze your glutes and raise your hips so that your body forms a straight line from shoulders to knees (B). Pause, then lower back to the starting position. That's 1 rep. Do 15.

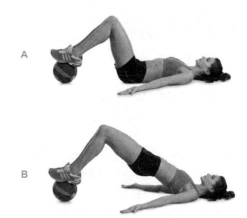

A

B

MEDICINE BALL TAP /

Place a medicine ball on the ground in front of you and lightly place your right foot on top of it, knee bent (A). Keeping your weight over your hips, switch feet so your left foot is on top of the ball (B); continue alternating as quickly as possible, picking up your knees and staying light on the balls of your feet. Do as many taps as you can in 1 minute.

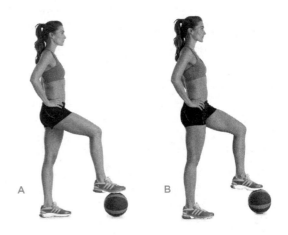

A

B

CIRCUIT 2

SQUAT WITH OVERHEAD
TOSS / Stand with your feet hip-width apart holding a medicine ball with both hands at chest height, elbows bent and close to your body. Sit your hips back and bend your knees to lower your body until your thighs are parallel to the floor (A). Pause, then press through your heels and explosively return to standing as you straighten your arms to press the ball toward the ceiling, releasing it overhead (B). Catch it, bending your knees to absorb the impact. Immediately lower into another rep. Do 15.

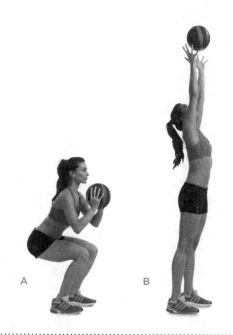

MEDICINE BALL DONKEY
KICK / Place the medicine ball on the floor and extend your legs behind you into a pushup position, feet wider than hip-width apart and hands on top of the ball. Keeping your core tight, bend your right knee toward your chest (A), pause, then press your heel up toward the ceiling, knee bent at 90 degrees (B). That's 1 rep. Immediately draw your knee back into your chest and continue for 10 reps, then switch sides and repeat.

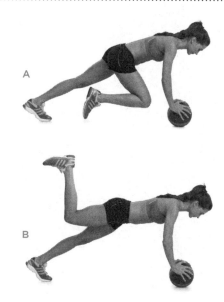

BENT-OVER ARM RAISE /

Holding a medicine ball with both hands, stand with your feet about shoulder-width apart, knees slightly bent; hinge forward at the hips to lower your torso toward the floor, keeping your back flat, arms hanging straight in line with your shoulders (A). Keeping your arms straight and without changing the position of your torso, brace your core and slowly raise the ball in front of you until your arms are on either side of your head (B). Pause, then slowly lower back to the starting position. That's 1 rep. Do 12 to 15.

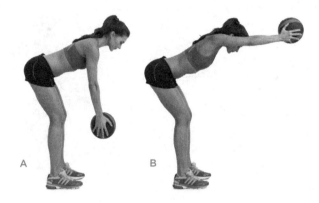

A

B

CIRCUIT 3

MEDICINE BALL SEATED TWIST WITH PRESS /

Holding a medicine ball with both hands, sit on the floor with your knees bent and feet flexed. Keep your back straight and hips facing forward as you twist your torso to the right and touch the weight to the floor next to you (A). Rotate back to the center and press the ball overhead (B), then lower it and rotate to the left (C). Reverse the movement to return to the starting position. That's 1 rep. Do 10.

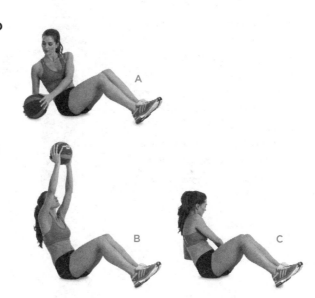

MEDICINE BALL BURPEE /

Stand with your feet slightly wider than shoulder-width apart, holding a medicine ball with both hands at your chest (A). Push your hips back, bend your knees, and squat down to place the ball on the floor, keeping both hands on the ball (B). Kick your legs back into a pushup position (C); quickly reverse the movement to return to standing. That's 1 rep. Do 15.

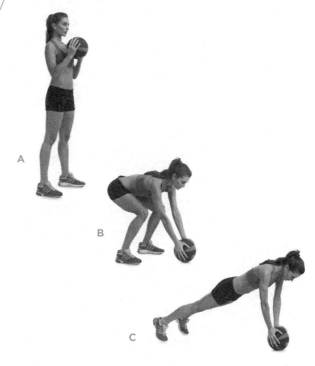

AROUND-THE-WORLD
LUNGE / Hold a medicine ball with both hands in front of your chest, feet shoulder-width apart (A). Take a big step to your left (B), lowering your body by pushing your hips back and bending your left knee as you circle the ball to the right and bring it over your left foot (C). Press through your left heel to return to the starting position. That's 1 rep. Repeat on the other side, and continue alternating for a total of 20 reps.

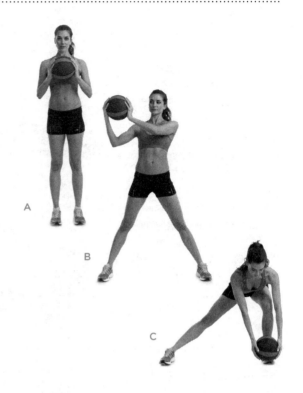

A

B

C

CABLE MACHINE

Unlike other gym machines that lock you into a fixed movement pattern, the cable machine allows for more functional movements so you can work your muscles from all angles with a greater range of motion. It also gives you a tough workout by keeping your muscles under constant tension, especially your core, which has to work overtime to stabilize your body each time you pull a cable. And it's a one-stop shop: You can get a killer head-to-toe workout without hopping around the gym. (If you don't have access to a cable machine, you can get a similar effect by using a resistance band to complete this workout. Simply anchor it to a sturdy object—like a banister—and then perform the exercises as instructed.)

This routine, created by Dan Trink, a strength coach and personal trainer at Peak Performance in New York City, is designed to build lean muscle and amp up your calorie burn during—and after—the workout. Complete 12 to 15 reps of each exercise, moving from one to the next without a break. Rest for 1 minute, then repeat the circuit three more times.

CABLE SQUAT TO ROW /
Grab a universal grip (a strap with two handles) in each hand and stand facing the cable machine, feet hip-width apart. Sit your hips back and bend your knees to lower your body toward the floor (A). As you stand, bend your elbows to row the handles to the sides of your chest (B). That's 1 rep.

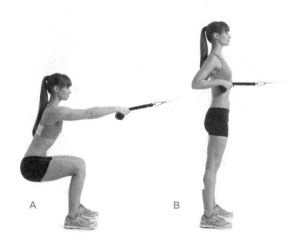

A   B

SINGLE-ARM CABLE CHEST PRESS / Using your left
hand, grab a handle attached at chest
height and face away from the machine,
elbow bent and palm down. Step your
left foot back into a split stance, knees
bent (A). Brace your abs and forcefully
press the handle forward (B). Do all
reps, then switch sides and repeat.

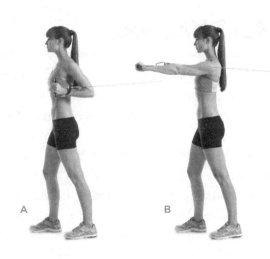

CABLE WOODCHOPPER /
Secure a handle at the highest point
and stand to the right of the
machine. Grab the handle with both
hands so your arms are extended
above your left shoulder, feet wide
and knees slightly bent (A). Keeping
your arms straight, pull the handle
across the front of your body to the
outside of your right thigh, shifting
your weight from your left foot to
your right (B). Slowly return to the
starting position. That's 1 rep. Do all
reps, then switch sides and repeat.

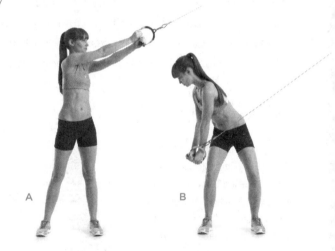

CABLE CORE PRESS /

Stand to the right of the cable machine and grab the handle (attached at chest height) with both hands at your chest (A). Keeping a tight core, press the handle directly out in front of you (B). Hold for 2 seconds, then return to the starting position. Complete all reps on that side, then turn to face the opposite direction and repeat.

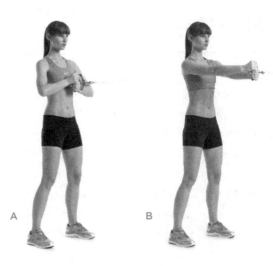

A

B

VALSLIDES

Staying fit on the road can be tough, I know. From packing logistics (running shoes take up precious carry-on room) and limited access to equipment or space, to just being super busy and tired—it can make fitting in a workout the last thing you want to do.

One of my solutions? Valslides. Created by the amazing Los Angeles–based trainer Valerie Waters, they're an affordable, portable replacement for slide boards that you might find in some gyms. They work on carpet, tile, hardwood floors—pretty much anything other than concrete—by reducing friction to create an unstable surface. Translation: They make basic moves far more difficult. And you can throw them in your gym bag, or, if you're like me, your carry-on. (I have taken very few trips without my Valslides.)

This simple routine is one of my go-tos when I need a fast, total-body workout on the road. Complete the prescribed number of reps for each exercise in order, moving from one to the next without rest. Rest for up to a minute, then repeat for a total of two or three circuits.

VALSLIDE PIKE / Get into a pushup position, hands directly under your shoulders and each foot on a Valslide. Your body should form a straight line from head to heels (A). Keeping your back flat and legs straight, brace your core and raise your hips to pull your feet toward your hands (B). Pause, then slowly return to the starting position. That's 1 rep. Do 12 to 15.

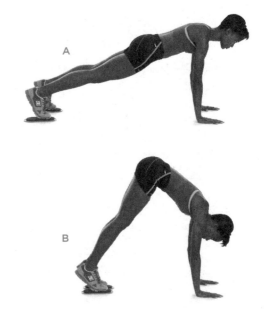

VALSLIDE CURTSY LUNGE /

Place your left foot on a Valslide and stand with your feet hip-width apart (A). In one motion, slide your left foot back and behind your right leg as you bend both knees to lower into a lunge (B). Press through your right heel to return to standing. That's 1 rep. Do 10 to 12, then switch legs and repeat.

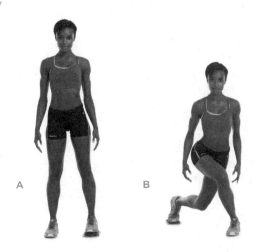

A

B

VALSLIDE PUSHUP /

Place your hands on the floor shoulder-width apart, your right hand on a Valslide, and extend both feet so that you're in a pushup position with your body forming a straight line from head to heels (A). Keeping your core tight, slide your right arm away from your left and bend both elbows to lower your body toward the ground as far as possible (B). Press through your left palm and pull your right hand back to the starting position. That's 1 rep. Do 6 to 8, then switch hands and repeat.

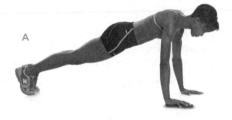

A

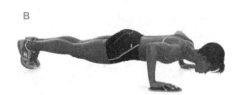

B

SINGLE-LEG VALSLIDE CURL /

Lie faceup on the floor with palms up, your left heel on a Valslide, and your right foot flat on the floor, knee bent (A). Squeeze your glutes and raise your hips off the ground. Bend your left knee and pull it toward your butt and in line with your right knee (B). Pause, then reverse the move to return to the starting position. That's 1 rep. Do 6 to 8, then switch legs and repeat.

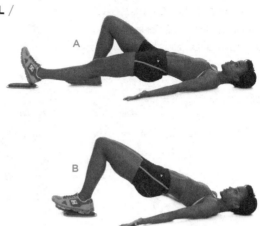

VALSLIDE ARM CIRCLE /

Place each hand on a Valslide directly under your shoulders and extend your feet behind you into a pushup position, your body forming a straight line from head to heels (A). Keeping your core tight and your hips parallel to the floor, slowly make a large clockwise circle with your right hand (B), returning it to the starting position under your shoulder. Repeat on the other side. That's 1 rep. Do 15.

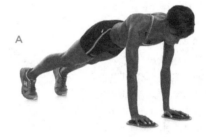

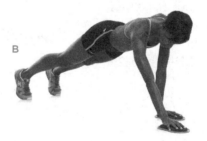

UPSIDE-DOWN SNOW
ANGEL

/ Get into a pushup position, hands directly under your shoulders and each foot on a Valslide. Your body should form a straight line from head to heels (A). Without dropping your hips, squeeze your glutes and slide your legs out to the sides as far as you can (B); pause, then slide them back together. That's 1 rep. Do 15.

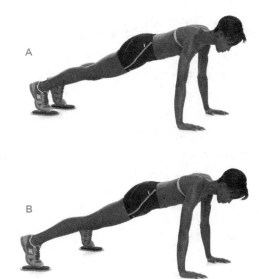

A

B

STABILITY BALL

Chances are, you've used a stability ball at some point in your workout history. It's a simple gym staple that continues to deliver top-notch results when used during basic core training. Case in point: Research shows that crunches atop a ball are approximately twice as effective as those done on the floor. But stop there and you're selling this multitasking tool short. A stability ball can be used as an effective tool for toning your entire body—not to mention improving flexibility, balance, posture, and coordination. Complete the prescribed reps of each of the following exercises in order, moving from one to the next with as little rest as possible. Rest for up to 1 minute, then repeat for a total of three sets.

STABILITY BALL LEG CURL /

Lie faceup on the floor and place your lower legs and heels on a stability ball. Extend your arms out to your sides at a 45-degree angle to your torso, palms facing up. Push your hips so that your body forms a straight line from your shoulders to your knees (A). Without pausing, pull your heels toward you and roll the ball as close as possible to your butt (B). Pause for a second or two, then reverse the motion by rolling the ball back until your body is in a straight line, to return to the starting position. That's 1 rep. Do 12 to 15.

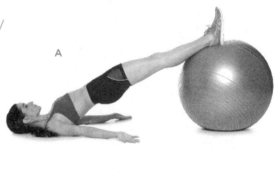

A

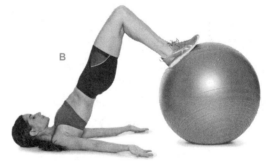

B

STABILITY BALL BACK EXTENSION

/ Lie facedown on a stability ball, hands behind your head, feet against a sturdy object like a wall (A). Squeeze your glutes and lift your torso up until your body forms a straight line (B). Hold for 1 or 2 seconds, then slowly lower your torso to return to the starting position. That's 1 rep. Do 12 to 15.

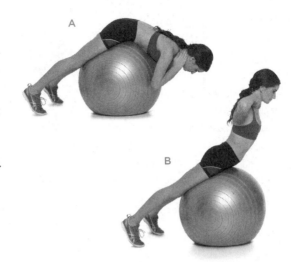

STABILITY BALL PIKE

/ Start in a pushup position with your arms straight, hands on the floor shoulder-width apart, and shins resting on top of a stability ball (A). Brace your abs and keep your legs straight as you raise your hips as high as you can toward the ceiling, drawing the ball toward your arms (B). Pause, then roll back to the starting position. That's 1 rep. Do 10 to 12.

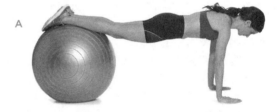

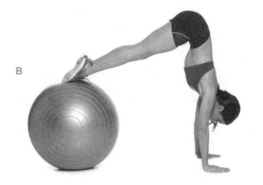

STABILITY BALL PUSHUP /

Start in a pushup position with your arms straight and slightly wider than your shoulders, with your legs extended and feet resting on top of a stability ball (A). Keeping your core braced and squeezing your glutes, bend your elbows to lower your body until your chest nearly touches the floor (B). Pause, then push yourself back to the starting position as quickly as possible. That's 1 rep. Do 8 to 10.

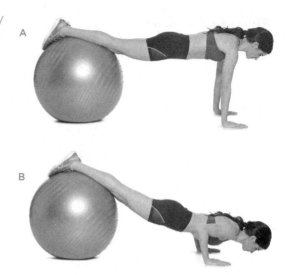

STABILITY BALL ARM CIRCLES /

Get into a forearm plank on top of the ball, your elbows underneath your shoulders and your feet about shoulder-width apart on the floor (A). Brace your core as you move the ball in a small clockwise circle using your elbows (B). Pause, then repeat in the opposite direction (C). That's 1 rep. Do 8 to 10.

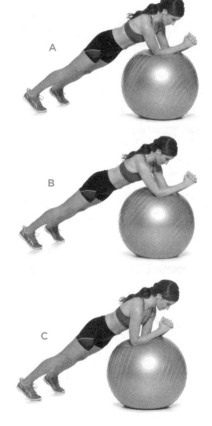

MINI BAND

Hands-down one of my favorite workout tools. This small, closed-loop band mobilizes your hips, activates your glutes, enhances your performance, and can challenge your stability and strength from head to toe. It can also help reduce your risk of injury: One study found that using the band during squats helps remind you to push your knees out, which can prevent injuries such as strains and tears to your knee's ligaments, such as your ACL. In addition to that, it's the size of an iPhone and cheaper than a morning latte. Complete the exercises in order, moving from one to the next without rest. Repeat for two or three sets.

BANDED GLUTE BRIDGE / Place a mini band just above your knees and lie faceup on the floor with your knees bent and feet flat on the floor (A). Squeeze your glutes as you lift your hips into the air so that your body forms one straight line from shoulders to knees, pushing outward against the band to keep your knees from touching (B). Pause, then lower your hips to return to the starting position. That's 1 rep. Do 15 to 20.

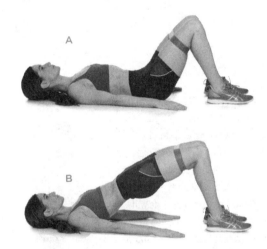

BANDED SQUAT / Place both legs inside a mini band and position the band just above your knees (A). With your arms outstretched and legs shoulder-width apart, push your hips back and bend your knees to lower into a squat (B). Keep your weight in your heels and focus on pushing your knees outward as you lower as far as you can go. Pause, then slowly push yourself back up to the starting position. That's 1 rep. Do 12 to 15.

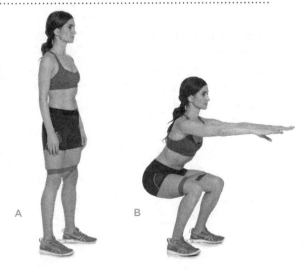

BANDED GLUTE KICKBACK /

Stand with a mini band around your ankles (A). Keeping your leg straight, squeeze your glutes and raise your right leg straight behind you, pressing through your left heel (B). Pause, then reverse the movement to return to the starting position. That's 1 rep. Do 12 to 15, then switch sides.

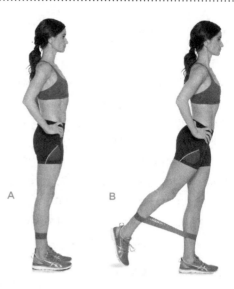

A   B

BANDED BOX WALK /

Place a mini band around your legs below your knees and stand with your feet hip-width apart, knees bent in an athletic stance (A). Keeping your core tight and chest upright, take one big step to the side with your right foot (B), followed by your left to return to the starting stance. Repeat 10 to 20 times. Then, step your right foot forward (C), followed by your left. Repeat 10 to 20 times. Repeat this pattern by taking 10 to 20 steps to the left, then 10 to 20 steps backward, until you've completed a "box" pattern.

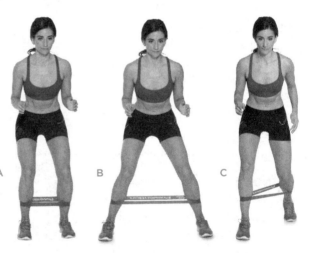

A   B   C

BANDED MOUNTAIN CLIMBER / Place a mini band around your feet and get into a pushup position, hands shoulder-width apart and legs extended so your body forms a straight line from head to heels (A). Brace your core and bend your left knee toward your chest (B). Pause, then slowly lower back to the starting position. Repeat on the other side. That's 1 rep. Do 10 to 12.

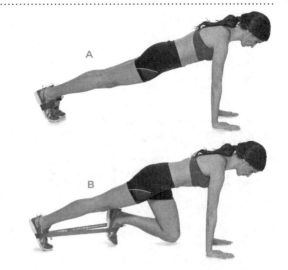

BANDED HAND TAP / Place a mini band around both wrists and get into a pushup position, hands under your shoulders and feet hip-width apart. There should be tension between your arms (A). Keeping your core engaged and maintaining a straight line from heels to head, bring your left hand next to your right (B), keeping your hips as still as possible. Reverse to return to start, and repeat on the other side. That's 1 rep. Do 12 to 15.

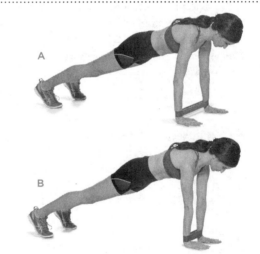

BANDED LYING LEG EXTENSION / Place a mini band around your calves and lie on your right side on the floor, with your right arm extended above your head, your left hand in front of you for support, and your feet stacked (A). Keeping your upper body still and legs straight, raise your left leg toward the ceiling (B); pause, then slowly lower back to the starting position. That's 1 rep. Do 12 to 15, then switch sides and repeat.

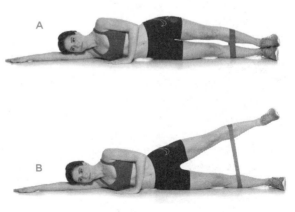

QUICK TIPS:
GROCERY SHOPPING

63 **Stock up on eggs.** They will keep in your refrigerator for 3 to 5 weeks. Older eggs are actually better for boiling because they're easier to peel. Want to know if your eggs are still good? Place one in a bowl of water. If it sinks, it's good; if it floats, it's time to toss 'em.

64 **Pick the better berries.** Adding blueberries instead of strawberries to your cereal will more than double your antioxidant intake.

65 **Fill up on avocado.** Avoid late-afternoon hunger pangs and the junk-snack run that goes with them by eating avocado—a tasty and versatile craving killer. Recent research published in *Nutrition Journal* found that adding half an avocado to people's lunches decreased their desire to eat over the next 3 hours by a whopping 40 percent. There are plenty of ways to incorporate it: Smash it on a piece of toast (duh), blend it into a green smoothie for a creamier texture, or wrap turkey around slices of it.

66 **Raise a glass of tomato juice.** More than just a base for your brunch cocktail, tomato juice is also a great recovery aid for your muscles. In one study, athletes who swapped their sports drink for tomato juice had less post-exercise inflammation than those who didn't—probably due to the unique blend of antioxidants in processed tomatoes.

67 **Add in some olive oil.** Put the breaks on your appetite with some healthy fat. Study participants who ate yogurt laced with olive oil had higher levels of serotonin, a hormone associated with fullness, than those who ate plain yogurt or yogurt spiked with other fats. Olive oil contains compounds that may slow glucose absorption, which can keep you feeling fuller for longer.

68 **Grab a basket.** Dashing into the store to pick up a few things? Skip the cart and choose a basket, instead. If you're limited to what you can carry, you're more likely to avoid impulse purchases. And head to the self-checkout line: One study found there was a 32 percent drop in impulse buys when participants used the fast lane.

69 **Look high and low.** Food manufacturers pay premium prices to ensure that their products sit on the middle shelf, where our eyes naturally fall as we walk down each aisle—and that fee is undoubtedly passed on to shoppers. When you hit up the soup, pasta, and packaged-goods aisles, you'll find better deals by shopping most heavily from the top and bottom shelves.

THE KEY TO SUCCESS: BE MOTIVATED BY WHAT YOU CAN DO, NOT DEFEATED BY WHAT YOU CAN'T DO.

FITNESS FIX

9 /

Your Weight- Loss Workout Plan

A FORGIVING AND FLEXIBLE fitness mentality—that is, doing any amount of exercise wherever and however possible—can be a productive and effective way to drop pounds. That's why this book is packed with routines that give you plenty of options, based on your schedule, your mood, and what type of equipment you have (or don't have).

But while freestyling your way through weekly workouts may offer variety, it can also make it harder to develop a consistent routine—especially for beginners. Without a set plan, a daily commitment to hit the gym can quickly slide. For many women, the problem is finding a program they can get into.

"The key to creating a maintainable fitness training plan is to address both our strength and cardio needs in short, simple, and effective workouts," says Robert dos Remedios, CSCS, strength and conditioning director at the College of the Canyons in Santa Clarita, California. He knows a thing or two about that winning combination. He, quite literally, wrote the book on it—it's called *Cardio Strength Training*. The two workouts you'll find in this chapter blend functional, balanced strength training in a circuit with short rest breaks to boost the cardiovascular benefits without compromising all-important lean muscle mass (which helps you burn even more calories after your workout). Oh yeah, and while many programs take about 45 minutes (sometimes more), you'll be done and on your way in 24 minutes.

Here's how to do it: Complete three routines each week on nonconsecutive days, alternating between Workout A and Workout B (so A-B-A during the first week, B-A-B during the second week, etc.). For each workout, start with the first exercise and complete as many reps as you can in 30 seconds, then rest for

30 seconds; continue to the next exercise and repeat this pattern until you've completed each move. That's 1 set. If you're a beginner (or it has been longer than 2 months since you've last exercised), repeat just one more time for a total of 2 sets. If you're more experienced, repeat three more times for a total of 4 sets. (It should take you about 20 minutes.)

After your sets, you'll have the option of doing a high-intensity, 4-minute "afterburn finisher." Think of it like extra credit, and aim to complete this exercise after most workouts—even if you're already tired. "It gives you a chance to stamp the exclamation point on a great workout—one more chance to throw an extra log on that metabolic furnace you're trying to ignite," says dos Remedios. It also helps you mentally push past your limits and test what your body is capable of achieving. They're super simple to complete: Do as many as you can in 20 seconds, then rest for 10 seconds. That's 1 set. Do 8 sets.

WEIGHT-LOSS WORKOUT A

DUMBBELL SKIER SWING /
Hold a pair of dumbbells and stand
with your feet hip-width apart. Push
your hips back and bring the weights
behind you (A), then quickly thrust
your hips forward and swing the
dumbbells to shoulder height,
squeezing your glutes and straightening your legs (B). That's 1 rep;
continue in a fluid, consistent
motion.

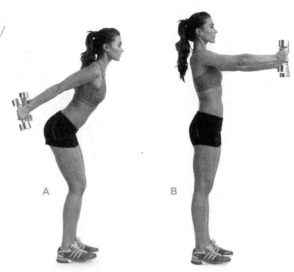

A   B

DUMBBELL GOBLET SQUAT /
Stand with your feet hip-width apart
and hold a dumbbell vertically in
front of your chest, with both hands
cupping the dumbbell head (A).
Push your hips back and bend your
knees to lower into a squat until your
thighs are parallel to the floor (B).
Push yourself back to the starting
position. That's 1 rep.

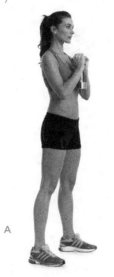
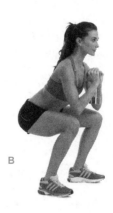

A   B

SUSPENDED PUSHUP /

Secure a TRX or other suspension system, face away from the anchor point with your feet shoulder-width apart, and hold both handles in front of your chest, arms extended (A). Bend your elbows to lower your chest toward the handles (performing a pushup), keeping a straight line from head to heels (B). Pause, then press back to the starting position. That's 1 rep.

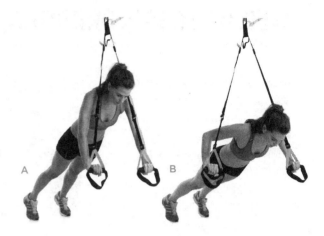

A   B

» *Don't have a suspension system like TRX? You can place your hands slightly wider than shoulder-width apart on a step or bench.*

DUMBBELL ROW /

Holding a dumbbell in each hand, stand with your feet hip-width apart, knees bent, arms hanging straight down, palms facing each other; bend forward to lower your torso toward the floor (A). Pull your shoulder blades together and row the weights toward your chest (B). Return to the starting position. That's 1 rep.

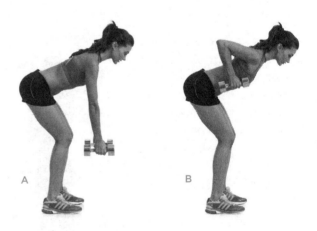

A   B

BODY SAW / Place your feet on Valslides and get into a pushup position, hands under your shoulders (A). (You can make the move easier by placing your forearms on the ground.) Keeping your body in a straight line from head to heels, push your feet away from you as far as you can (B). Pull back to the starting position, pressing through your palms. That's 1 rep.

» *No Valslides? You can also use small towels or even paper plates in their place.*

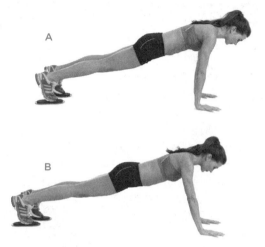

A

B

FINISHER » JUMP ROPE / Grab the handles of a jump rope, starting with the rope behind you. Keeping your body upright and elbows close, make small circles with your wrists to swing the rope over your head. Jump off the floor as the rope passes under your feet, and land softly on the balls of your feet. Continue as quickly as possible.

WEIGHT-LOSS WORKOUT B

JUMP SQUAT / Standing with your feet hip-width apart and keeping your chest up and core tight, sit your hips back to lower into a squat, raising your arms in front of you at shoulder height (A). Press through your heels to jump as high as you can off the ground, swinging your arms behind you (B). That's 1 rep. Land softly and immediately lower into your next squat.

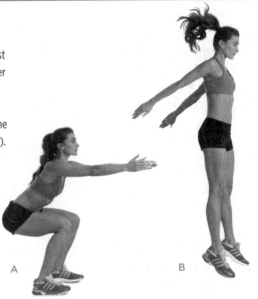

WALKING LUNGE / Stand with your feet hip-width apart, hands on your hips (A). Step forward with your left leg and lower your body until both knees are bent 90 degrees (B). Press through your left heel and bring your right foot forward as you return to standing. That's 1 rep. Repeat on the other side and continue alternating.

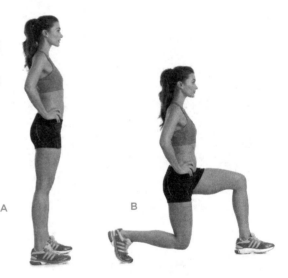

DUMBBELL PUSH PRESS /

Hold a pair of dumbbells at shoulder height, palms facing each other, feet hip-width apart. Bend your knees slightly (A), then stand and press the dumbbells overhead, straightening your arms completely (B). That's 1 rep.

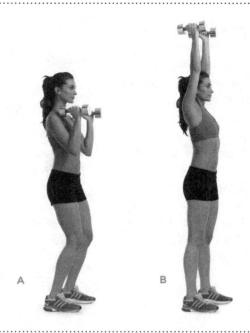

SUSPENDED ROW / Secure

a TRX or other suspension system and face the anchor point, holding both handles in front of your chest, arms straight, feet shoulder-width apart (A). Keep your shoulders back and bend your elbows to pull your body toward the anchor point (B). Pause, then slowly return to the starting position. That's 1 rep.

» You can adjust the level of difficulty of this move by changing where you place your feet. As you walk your feet farther away from you, you will be pulling a higher percentage of your own body weight. (If you don't have a TRX, you can use a squat rack or Smith machine.)

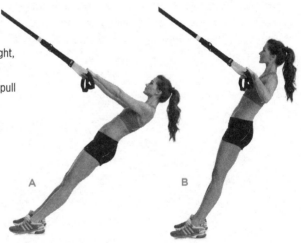

ALTERNATING BAND ROTATIONS / Stand facing a resistance band (secured a few feet away from you at chest height) and grab the handle with both hands, then step away until you feel tension (A). Keeping your arms completely straight, brace your core and pull the handle to the right while rotating your hips and shoulders (B). Pause, then return to the starting position. That's 1 rep. Repeat on the left side and continue alternating.

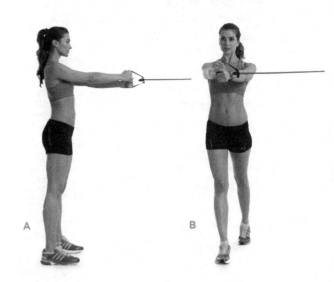

A

B

FINISHER » MOUNTAIN CLIMBER / Start at the top of a pushup position, with your body forming a straight line from head to heels. Keeping your abs braced and back flat, pick up your right foot and bend your knee toward your chest. Return to the starting position and repeat with the other foot; continue alternating. (Refer to the photos on page 92.)

KEEP MAKING PROGRESS

There's no limit to how long you can follow the program—and you'll never hit a plateau. How's that possible? "It's very easy to quantify your results and see progress," says Robert dos Remedios, CSCS, strength and conditioning director at the College of the Canyons. For example, after a few weeks of doing squat jumps, you will start to see a pattern in how many reps you can complete in 30 seconds. "As you get stronger and fitter, this number will increase. You can add intensity by either increasing the reps or the load—say, by using light dumbbells."

The amount of weight you should use will vary from person to person, but as a general rule, dos Remedios recommends using a tempo of 2 seconds per rep as a guide. So if you're doing, let's say, goblet squats, you should be getting in around 15 reps in 30 seconds. If you're not even close to this number, decrease your weight and try to pick up the pace. If you're busting out more like 20 reps, you should grab some heavier dumbbells. Regardless of how many pounds you're hoisting, you should be struggling to finish the last few reps (especially toward the end of the circuit), but without losing proper form.

QUICK TIPS:
EATING FOR WEIGHT LOSS

70 **Keep that caffeine habit.** Sip about 270 milligrams of caffeine—roughly the amount in a tall Starbucks coffee—before your workout to help raise the number of calories you torch afterward. When cyclists sipped espresso an hour before a ride, their resting metabolism—the number of calories they burned while not working out—leaped by 15 percent post-ride.

71 **Pack on the protein.** When you drop pounds, some of what you shed is calorie-burning muscle—a loss that can slow your metabolism. One fix: Double your protein. Study participants who downed twice the recommended daily allowance lost the same amount of weight—but much less muscle—as those who ate the RDA. Aim for 1.5 grams per 2 pounds of body weight per day to reap the results.

72 **Stack your day.** A study in the journal *Obesity* found that women who ate a 700-calorie breakfast and a 200-calorie dinner shed more than twice as much weight over 12 weeks as those whose meal sizes were reversed. Your body clock is linked to hormone dips that rev metabolism in the morning and leave it feeling sluggish at night, say study authors.

73 **Drop the guilt.** Twenty-seven percent of people associated chocolate cake with guilt. In a study from the University of Canterbury, those who felt bad about eating it were less likely to maintain their weight over a year and a half compared with the 73 percent of people who associate the dessert with celebration.

74 **Be wary of white bread.** Limit your intake of white bread to less than 120 grams (four or five slices) a week. People are 40 percent more likely to be overweight if white bread is the only bread they eat, according to Spanish researchers.

75 **Power up with protein.** Start your day with eggs and ham. Having a larger serving of protein at breakfast makes you less likely to over-eat for the rest of the day, say researchers. Shoot for at least 20 grams.

76 **Cut back on carbs.** It's one of the most reli-able strategies for short-term weight loss. Dutch researchers found that eating one carb-free meal a day over a 2-week period can increase your met-abolic rate by 81 calories per day. The key is making the meal about 70 percent protein and, of course, zero carbs. Watch for sneaky carb sources like milk, sausages, and barbecue sauce, just to name a few.

77 **Replace, don't remove.** Cutting calo-ries too drastically can feel taxing, mentally and physi-cally. Instead, make one tweak during each meal to get more nutrients like healthy fats, fiber, and protein into your diet. It's as simple as sprin-kling your yogurt with flax-seed instead of granola at breakfast or adding a handful of fresh spinach to your pasta sauce at dinner.

78 **Dine in.** It should come as no surprise that weekends are the most popu-lar days for dining out, according to the National Restaurant Association. But research has also found that eating dinner out adds 144 calories to your daily intake. It may not seem like a lot, but if you also ate out for lunch, that's another 158 calories—plus, any away-from-home snacks tack on about 107 calories each.

TRUST THE PROCESS. EMBRACE THE JOURNEY.

FITNESS FIX

10 /

Run
Your
Butt Off

EVEN THOUGH I'M STRESSING short-and-sweet workouts and that you don't need a full-fledged cardio plan, I know some of you don't want to ditch your running routine. I get it. That's why I've included this simple but efficient 8-week weight-loss program created by Andrew Kastor, head coach at Mammoth Track Club in Mammoth Lakes, California (and, yes, husband of three-time Olympian Deena Kastor). Good news: You don't need to log more than one long run a week (meaning 30 minutes or more). This sustained effort will improve your endurance by increasing your heart's capacity and strengthening ligaments and tendons so you feel stronger during your short runs.

GET BACK ON THE ROAD

Like I've said, running is not a requirement for fat loss; however, it is an incredibly accessible tool (no equipment required but you and your sneakers!). But if you're a beginning runner (or it's been 6 months or longer since you ran anything over a mile), ramping up your mileage or speed too quickly can book you an express ticket back to the sidelines.

The best thing you can do is start out slowly—really slowly. Easing into it helps your muscles get used to the impact of running and helps your mind get used to the effort. Use this run/walk program three times a week (on nonconsecutive days). Begin and end each session with a 5-minute warmup walk. Repeat a week if you don't feel ready to move up. The sign that you're ready to start tacking on more mileage (and eventually, speed): You can run consistently for at least 30 minutes.

WEEK 1: Run 2 minutes, walk 3 minutes; repeat 6 times.
WEEK 2: Run 3 minutes, walk 3 minutes; repeat 5 times.
WEEK 3: Run 5 minutes, walk 2 minutes; repeat 4 times.
WEEK 4: Run 7 minutes, walk 3 minutes; repeat 4 times.
WEEK 5: Run 8 minutes, walk 2 minutes; repeat 3 times.
WEEK 6: Run 9 minutes, walk 1 minute; repeat 3 times.
WEEK 7: Run 30 minutes.

READY TO RUN

Use these as a guide to follow the 8-week beginner and experienced running programs on the following pages.

CROSS-TRAINING (XT)

Choose another form of low- to moderate-intensity aerobic exercise (that is, swimming, easy hiking, cycling, elliptical machine, kick boxing)

STRENGTH

Should be total body or focused on core and legs. Use any workout in this book. Note: This is in addition to the time shown on the calendar for cross training or running.

MAIN RUN

Beginners should follow a 4-minute easy run/1-minute walk pattern each week, repeating for the prescribed duration. In the experienced plan, choose the initial starting duration based on your current mileage, then maintain a steady-state run, walking only when necessary.

INTERVALS

After a 10-minute warmup at an easy pace, run hard (nearly all-out effort) for 30 seconds, then slow down to recover (jogging or walking) for 60 seconds. Repeat for the prescribed number of sets. Finish with a 10-minute cooldown.

HILLS

After a 10-minute warmup at an easy pace, find a gentle hill (or use up to 5 percent incline on a treadmill), and run hard for 10 seconds, then walk down or recover for up to 60. Repeat for the prescribed number of sets. Finish with a 10-minute cooldown.

WATCH YOUR STEP

Just like with strength training, proper form during aerobic exercise is crucial. Sharpen your step with these simple form pointers.

FAST FEET
Take quick, short steps instead of longer strides, which can hurt your lower back and tire you out. Your feet should land under your center of gravity, not out in front of you.

SOFT STEPS
Land lightly between your heel and midfoot, and let your foot roll smoothly forward. Push off with your toes.

HEAD UP
Look ahead and scan the horizon to prevent slouching (unless you're running on a trail or other bumpy surface).

STRAIGHT SWING
Relax your arms and bend them about 90 degrees, letting them swing front to back (not across your midline) between waist and lower-chest level. Keep your hands loose—think about lightly holding a piece of paper between your thumb and pointer finger.

LEAN IN
Lean forward from your hips to maintain momentum without sacrificing your posture. (To get the approximate feel, stand still on both feet, then shift your weight toward the balls of your feet without lifting your heels.)

PROUD CHEST
Keep your chest lifted, shoulders stretching down your back. Imagine there is a string attached to your sternum pulling you upward as you run.

BEGINNER / WEEKS 1–8

	MONDAY	TUESDAY	WEDNESDAY	THURSDAY	FRIDAY	SATURDAY	SUNDAY
1	XT + Strength (20–30 min)	Interval (x6)	Off	Hills (optional) (x4)	XT + Strength (20–30 min)	Main Run (15 min)	Off
2	XT + Strength (20–30 min)	Interval (x6)	Off	Hills (optional) (x5)	XT + Strength (20–30 min)	Main Run (20 min)	Off
3	XT + Strength (20–30 min)	Interval (x7)	Off	Hills (optional) (x6)	XT + Strength (20–30 min)	Main Run (25 min)	Off
4	XT + Strength (20–30 min)	Interval (x7)	Off	Hills (optional) (x7)	XT + Strength (20–30 min)	Main Run (30 min)	Off
5	XT + Strength (20–30 min)	Interval (x6)	Off	Hills (optional) (x5)	XT + Strength (20–30 min)	Main Run (30–60 min)	Off
6	XT + Strength (20–30 min)	Interval (x7)	Off	Hills (optional) (x6)	XT + Strength (20–30 min)	Main Run (35–65 min)	Off
7	XT + Strength (20–30 min)	Interval (x8)	Off	Hills (optional) (x7)	XT + Strength (20–30 min)	Main Run (40–70 min)	Off
8	XT + Strength (20–30 min)	Interval (x8)	Off	Hills (optional) (x8)	XT + Strength (20–30 min)	Main Run (45–75 min)	Off

EXPERIENCED / WEEKS 1-8

	MONDAY	TUESDAY	WEDNESDAY	THURSDAY	FRIDAY	SATURDAY	SUNDAY
1	XT + Strength (20–30 min)	Interval (x8)	Off	Hills (optional) (x6)	Run (optional) + Strength (20–30 min)	Main Run (30–60 min)	Off
2	XT + Strength (20–30 min)	Interval (x9)	Off	Hills (optional) (x7)	Run (optional) + Strength (20–30 min)	Main Run (35–65 min)	Off
3	XT + Strength (20–30 min)	Interval (x10)	Off	Hills (x8)	Run (optional) + Strength (20–30 min)	Main Run (40–70 min)	Off
4	XT + Strength (20–30 min)	Interval (x11)	Off	Hills (x9)	Run (optional) + Strength (20–30 min)	Main Run (45–75 min)	Off
5	Run + Strength (20–30 min)	Interval (x9)	Off	Hills (x7)	Run (optional) + Strength (20–30 min)	Main Run (30–60 min)	Off
6	Run + Strength (20–30 min)	Interval (x10)	Off	Hills (x8)	Run (optional) + Strength (20–30 min)	Main Run (35–65 min)	Off
7	Run + Strength (20–30 min)	Interval (x11)	Off	Hills (x9)	Run (optional) + Strength (20–30 min)	Main Run (40–70 min)	Off
8	Run + Strength (20–30 min)	Interval (x12)	Off	Hills (x10)	Run (optional) + Strength (20–30 min)	Main Run (45–75 min)	Off

QUICK TIPS:
CARDIO

79 **Even out your effort.** Most people take an attack-and-conquer approach to hills, but hammering as hard as possible can cause you to burn out quickly. Instead, climb up at the same *perceived effort* (rather than pace) as your flat-terrain running. As you descend the hill, keep an even effort by speeding up.

80 **Run those hills.** Hill workouts increase your speed and power, improve your stamina, prevent overuse injuries by engaging different muscles, and give you a gorgeous set of gams. The icing on the cake: For each degree of incline, experts say you can count on at least a 10 percent increase in calories burned. So running up a 5 percent grade—a gentle hill—will burn 50 percent more calories than running on a totally flat surface for the same amount of time.

81 **Start with a small incline and build.** Don't jump straight to a 5 percent incline on the treadmill—you'll hate it and never want to do it again. Start with a 2 to 3 percent incline. If you're outdoors, look for a gradual hill or incline—one that challenges you but doesn't force you to stop or walk. It should feel tough but manageable.

82 **Embrace a few well-deserved walking breaks.** Taking short walk breaks may feel like "cheating," but it can help you run farther, burn more calories, and sidestep injury. So whether you're working up to 3 miles or training for a long-distance event, walking now and then can serve as a useful tool to build up your mileage and endurance. The key is making sure you're stopping only two or three times during a 30-minute run, for about 1 minute each time.

83 **Stretch after cardio sessions.** Cramming in your cardio? Stretch after—not before—to go farther and faster, report Florida State University researchers. Subjects who didn't loosen up prior to a 30-minute treadmill run logged an extra 220 yards compared with those who stretched for more than 15 minutes beforehand. Normally, muscle fibers are like tight rubber bands, springing your legs off the ground faster so your feet move quicker. Stretching lengthens these fibers, making them less elastic and slower to react. Instead, study authors recommend warming up with a 5- to 10-minute jog or brisk walk.

84 Strengthen your hips. You may think you have "bad knees" from running, but research is pointing to weak hip muscles as the culprit behind running-related injuries, according to a review in *Sports Health: A Multidisciplinary Approach*. Weak hips change your normal ankle and knee alignment when you jog, which stresses tissues unnaturally. A simple exercise to help improve hip strength and mobility: leg circles. Lie on your back and raise one leg 6 inches off the ground, keeping your knee straight. Slowly move your

leg clockwise in a small circle; do 10 circles in each direction, then switch legs and repeat. Roll onto your side, with your hips stacked on top of each other, and repeat the pattern (circling the leg forward and then backward); roll onto your other side and repeat.

85 Swim yourself slim. Get more from your cross-training by swimming. Water is about 800 times thicker than air. Translation: Pool training requires your muscles to push continuously against its resistance, building strength and endurance.

86 Add a weighted vest. Wearing a weighted vest can help you burn more calories. In a recent study, women who wore one while walking burned up to 12 percent more calories than those who went vestless. To amp up your walk or run, start with a vest that's 3 to 5 percent of your weight to minimize your risk.

CHASING DREAMS IS THE BEST KIND OF CARDIO.

FITNESS FIX

11 / What's Cooking?

YOU MAY HAVE HEARD the saying, "Abs are made in the kitchen." Which is true—as long as you're the one doing the cooking.

In 2009, Americans began spending more money on eating out than preparing meals at home. In fact, total food dollars spent on out-of-home foods have increased 97 percent over the past 40 years. People aren't hitting up the drive-thru for their health: They do it because of the convenience. In fact, when researchers at the University of Minnesota School of Public Health surveyed adults about their attitudes toward fast foods, there was no link between frequency of fast-food intake and perceived healthfulness of fast food; however, frequency of intake was significantly associated with perceived convenience and a dislike of cooking.

I've been there. After a hectic day, when I know I don't have anything prepped or planned at home, it feels infinitely easier to order takeout. But here's the thing: For all the points eating out scores for convenience, it loses ten times as many for a lack of calorie control. Experts estimate that eating at a restaurant increases your total calorie intake by 36 percent compared to eating at home. What's worse, you probably don't have a clue how many calories your entrée really contains: According to recent data from the University of Arkansas, the average diner underestimates each meal by up to 600 calories. Still need more reasons to eat in? Ninety-six percent of entrées sold in American chain restaurants contain more than one-third of the USDA's daily recommendations for calories, sodium, and total or saturated fat. What's more, people who regularly ate fast food over 6 years were 41 percent more likely to become depressed than those who avoided the greasy grub, reports the journal *Public Health Nutrition*. Scientists believe the high trans fats content in fast foods may interfere with the brain's ability to produce certain mood-stabilizing neurotransmitters. For your physical and mental health, limit drive-thru trips and eat more fruits and vegetables.

Don't get obsessed over every little detail. Just like with exercise, the first step is developing consistency through smaller efforts. It's not about making gourmet meals or following some tight set of diet guidelines. Just start cooking. That alone will help, trust me. Cook at home just 3 days a week and you could lose a pound a week. And the benefits go beyond the scale: People who cook often have a healthier relationship with food and are more likely to be satisfied by what they eat. In fact, researchers have found that women who take a forward-thinking approach to food and cooking (meaning they try new recipes, plan meals, and shop with a list) have a higher intake of vegetables.

Cutting back on takeout doesn't mean you have to eat a bowl of cereal for dinner every night. All you need to know to prepare delicious, calorie-conscious meals at home are a few simple cooking and prepping methods.

ROASTING

Roasting caramelizes the sugars in meats and vegetables, developing their natural sweetness, so it's a great way to enhance the flavor of everything from whole chicken and pork roast to vegetables (like potatoes, Brussels sprouts, and squash) and fatty fish like salmon—without adding calories. And the best part of roasting? Very little prep is required. Just preheat the oven to 400°F. Lightly coat the ingredients with olive oil and season with salt, pepper, and your favorite dried herbs. Use a meat thermometer to determine when meats are done. Vegetables are ready when they start to brown on the outside and are tender on the inside, usually 35 to 40 minutes. (Give them a quick toss after about 20 minutes.)

SAUTÉING

This quick-cooking technique involves constantly tossing or stirring the food with a tablespoon or two of oil or butter over high heat. It preserves the natural flavors, textures, and colors of foods and is a great cooking method for naturally tender cuts of meat (such as beef tenderloin, fish fillets, or chicken breast) and quick-cooking vegetables (such as asparagus, peppers, broccoli, onions, sugar snap peas, and mushrooms). When chopping for a sauté, cut everything into uniform pieces so your food cooks at the same rate. Then add just enough oil to coat the skillet and place it over medium-high heat for a minute or two. Before adding all the ingredients, test the heat level with a single piece; it should sizzle when it hits the skillet. (If you add the food before the skillet and oil are hot enough, the food will release its liquid and your dish will turn out soggy.) Add your ingredients to the skillet and cook over medium-high heat, tossing frequently, until meats are cooked through and veggies are tender-crisp. If you're cooking a mix of foods, brown your meat first, then add aromatics (garlic, onions) and vegetables.

BROILING

By putting food directly under exposed high heat (broiling), you can give it a crispy texture on the outside while keeping it moist and juicy inside—all without adding much oil or fat. Use this method when cooking thin cuts of meat or fish that will cook quickly and taste great with a golden-brown exterior—think flank or skirt steaks, lamb or pork chops, and all kinds of fish.

All meat needs is a dash of salt and freshly ground pepper; drizzle fish with olive oil and lemon juice. Set the broiler to high; if your oven doesn't have a built-in broiler, adjust your top oven rack so that it is about 8 inches from the top heating element. The thickness of the cut and how well-done you like your meat will determine how long to leave it in—ranging from 3 minutes per side for a thin, rare steak to 9 minutes per side for a thick, well-done one.

SPIRALIZING

A few years ago, I started hearing people talking more and more about "zoodles," or zucchini noodles. I was skeptical. How could spiralized vegetables actually taste like noodles? This had to be one of those things people on diets try to convince themselves "tastes just like the real thing," right? Then my parents got me one for Christmas. Now I'm not someone to fawn over kitchen appliances, but I can say without hesitation that this one tool has completely changed the way I eat—and the way I think about preparing quick, easy, nutritious meals.

You see, I'm not someone who craves salads all the time, but I am someone who's always looking for ways to fit more fresh produce into my diet. This one tool has honestly made the biggest impact on my intake. Consider that a woman in her forties should aim to consume $2\frac{1}{2}$ cups of vegetables a day. She can check that entire total off with just one bowl of zucchini noodles. But it goes far beyond zucchini: apples, beets, butternut squash, carrots, jicama, parsnip, and sweet potatoes can all be spiralized and used to add more veggies to everything from frittatas and soups to nachos and desserts.

You can also store prepared vegetable noodles in the fridge or freezer for even easier plan-ahead meals: Just line an airtight glass or plastic container with paper towels and seal the noodles inside; they'll stay fresh for 4 to 5 days. (After that they'll start to stiffen and lose flavor.)

BLENDING

Assemble the recommended nine servings of fruits and vegetables on your kitchen counter, and the prospect of fitting them into 24 hours may feel next to impossible. Blend them into an ice-cold smoothie, however, and it's suddenly much less daunting. This is just one reason why I don't see this trend going anywhere anytime soon. Smoothies are a supersimple—not to mention portable and delicious—way to get more fruits and vegetables (yes, vegetables!) into your daily diet.

But it doesn't stop at smoothies. Bored with salad? Soup can be an equally filling and slimming meal: According to a study published in the journal *Physiology & Behavior,* people consumed the fewest calories on days when they ate soup rather than the same ingredients in solid form. Another study published in *Appetite* found that people who started lunch with vegetable soup ended up eating 20 percent less than those who skipped the soup. And while creamy, rich soups tend to be high in calories and fat when you eat them at restaurants, you can blend rich, creamy consistency soups at home for a fraction of the caloric cost. Blenders can also be used to whip together fruit-and-veggie–rich sorbets, sauces, and dips.

SLOW COOKING

This one's really as easy as it gets, people. Most slow cooker recipes are inherently easy and require very little prep work; simply toss all the ingredients in, turn it on, and let it do the rest. It's the only appliance that cooks for you—safely—while you're at work or in bed or out doing anything other than slaving away in the kitchen, which is why it's practically magic for anyone who's trying to eat healthier but doesn't have a lot of free time.

Another big perk? Inexpensive cuts of meat also happen to possess an inordinate amount of flavor, but to enjoy it, you first need to break down all the connective tissue in the meat. Steady, low temperatures do it best, which is why slow cookers are so useful: Dump a bunch of inexpensive meat and vegetables in, cover with your choice of liquid (from red wine and vinegar to beef or chicken stock), press On, and disappear for 8 hours. Slow cookers also offer an effortless way to cook dried beans: Simply cover dried beans with plenty of water, add a few cloves of garlic or bay leaves (for enhanced flavor), and cook on low for 4 hours. No more soaking overnight!

HIDE YOUR VEGGIES!

Could the same trick that got you to eat your peas when you were a kid help you lose weight now? Penn State researchers think so. When blended or pureed vegetables were sneaked into three daily meals, study subjects ate nearly 360 fewer calories than when they were given the regular versions. (That could add up to a 3-pound loss in 1 month!) Break out your blender or food processor and make these swaps.

» **PASTA SALAD** / Skip the ½ cup mayo and add ½ cup pureed roasted peppers instead; you'll save 435 calories.

» **VEGGIE DIP** / Skip ¼ cup of the sour cream and add ½ cup of spinach, cooked, strained, and pureed; you'll save 79 calories.

» **BROWNIE MIX** / Skip the oil and add ½ cup of pureed beets and 1 can (15.5 ounces) of black beans, pureed; you'll save 469 calories.

» **CHOWDER** / Skip 1 cup of cream and add 2 cups of sweet corn, pureed; you'll save 556 calories.

QUICK TIPS:
VEGETABLES

87 **Season your eggplant.** Salt slices and let them sit for 20 minutes, then squeeze and pat dry. Salt draws out the bitter juice and keeps the spongy flesh from absorbing too much oil during cooking.

88 **Put your onions on ice.** To avoid crying, freeze the onion for 10 minutes. Doing so prevents the release of the enzymes that irritate your eyes. And when sautéing onions, add a pinch of baking soda. It speeds browning and cuts cooking time practically in half.

89 **Skin a tomato in a second.** Cut a small X into the skin. Drop the tomato into boiling water and wait 15 seconds; fish it out with a slotted spoon and then drop it into ice water. The skin will slide right off.

90 **Steam simply.** The two biggest mistakes people make when microwaving vegetables are dousing them with too much water and cooking them way too long. Washing veggies and not drying them will add just enough water. Place them in a microwavable dish with the lid slightly ajar. As for cooking times, a good starting point is 1 minute for every cup of tender produce, like fresh spinach and asparagus, and 3 minutes for every cup of heartier fresh vegetables, such as broccoli and carrots. After the initial time is up, hit the "add 30 seconds" button until your veggies are cooked the way you like them.

91 **Soak and spin.** Soak bitter greens, like arugula and kale, in a bowl of ice water in the fridge for about an hour to cut their bitterness. Run the leaves through your salad spinner several times with a paper towel to get them nice and dry and crisp. Want a more flavorful salad? Make sure the lettuce is completely dry; it helps the dressing stick.

92 **Roast everything.** When you're not sure what to do with an exotic veggie, roast it! Everything from sunchokes to rutabaga tastes great tossed with a little olive oil, seasoned with salt and pepper, and cooked in the oven at 400°F until tender.

93 **Sauté with broth.** It's healthier than using oil or butter, and you'll have crispy, seasoned vegetables without using heated, oxidized oil (which can cause free-radical damage in your body). Pour in just enough broth to cover the bottom of the pan, and cook, lid on, until tender.

94 **Watch out for hazardous hot peppers.** Wear gloves when handling extremely hot peppers; their oils burn like crazy, and soap and water won't always remove them.

FOCUS ON PROGRESS, NOT PERFECTION.

FITNESS FIX

12/

Meal
Prep
Made
Simple

YOU KNOW THOSE PERCEIVED roadblocks to healthy eating—that it's too expensive, too time-consuming, too complicated, too strict, or too bland and boring? I think a lot of them stem from our country's deep-rooted obsession with being on a diet. What foods are in, what foods are out, the complicated meal plans and super-pricey shopping lists. It's no wonder that how to eat and lose or maintain weight is an area where people feel desperate—and why people will try anything that promises to help them avoid the potential pitfalls. People tend to go on diets because they give us all the answers. Diets offer us a cheat sheet of sorts. We don't have to come up with recipe ideas, we don't have to look up a ton of nutrition information. We just buy what they tell us to and eat it. But while, yes, adherence to a diet program can be a very useful tool, especially in the beginning, it's just another short-term fix. To establish a life-long relationship with healthy eating, you've got to take some of the control back into your own hands.

While I'm not a dietician, I've talked to enough experts to know one thing: There are a million different diets that *can* work. But the diet you choose has to be one that works for you. (As in, you could see yourself following it *for the rest of your life*.) Like I said earlier, when people do (or in this case, eat) things that are fast, easy, and enjoyable, they're more likely to repeat that behavior. The more regular those habits become, the more the number on the scale will shift. Thinking ahead and stocking your home with some basic healthy ingredients are the first steps toward making that happen.

There are a lot of different ways to do meal prep, and everyone is going to be different based on their personal tastes and situations (say, if you're a vegan

The ingredients listed in this chapter—just like the ingredients listed in the majority of recipes you read—aren't set in stone. If you have a bag of unused mushrooms in the fridge but the recipe calls for eggplant, chances are the 'shrooms will do just fine. Don't want to spend $3 on a bunch of celery just to use a single stalk? Omit it. You like pork chops more than chicken breast? Switch it. The point is, once you understand the basic techniques and have an idea of what tastes good together, the possibility for creation in the kitchen is infinite.

versus someone who prefers lots of red meat, or if you're cooking for one or for a family of five). Some women find it helpful to spend a day making—and pre-portioning out—all of their meals for the week. That works. If you're someone who tends to get bored eating the same thing every day (like me), take a slightly looser approach: Think of your fridge as an at-home Chipotle. Prepare big batches of the big categories—a healthy grain or legume, one or two lean proteins, and a few different varieties of produce. For example: On a Sunday, I might make a big batch of brown rice, cook a pound of ground turkey mixed with black beans and tomatoes, and spiralize a few different veggies (a sweet potato, a few big carrots, a few zucchini). I put them all in separate airtight storage containers in my fridge; I'll also make sure to have a dozen eggs, a bag of fresh spinach, and a few "toppings" (usually a salsa or simple sauce, some kind of cheese, and an avocado). Boom. With this simple group of ingredients prepped and ready to go, I can mix and match endless healthy meal combinations throughout the week—without ever having to stress over the question, "What am I going to eat today?"

What I am proposing isn't a diet program. It's a way to shift your mindset about eating so that you can completely transform your waistline—and your life. Smart nutrition is crucial, but as you'll see on the following pages, that doesn't mean it has to be complicated. Consider this: If you cut out just 96 calories from your daily diet, you'll be 10 pounds lighter 1 year from today—and that's *without* exercise or any strict diet programs. So start with the big picture: Add some of these power foods to your grocery list each week. Just like with exercise, once you reach a point where planning ahead, cooking at home, and incorporating healthy ingredients become second nature, you can continue to step up your game—say, by starting to focus more specifically on your macronutrient breakdown and portion sizes to facilitate better fat-loss results or by asking your doctor if there are any vitamins or nutrients you could benefit from adding into your diet.

PROTEIN

Did you know that anywhere between 10 and 30 percent of the calories you burn every day get burned by the simple act of eating and digesting food? Yep, it's true. Also true: Your body uses almost twice as many calories digesting protein as it does fats and carbohydrates. What's more, substituting meat, fish, dairy, and nuts for carbs can help reduce the amount of fat around your middle. Researchers at McMaster University in Hamilton, Ontario, assessed the diets of 617 people and discovered that when they exchanged carbohydrates in favor of an equal amount of protein, they reduced overall belly fat.

MEAT

Not all protein is created equal. The healthiest cuts? Skinless, white chicken breast; lean turkey; pork tenderloin; and bison or beef top sirloin. That's not to say that options like grass-fed ground beef, beef flank, and beef T-bone are off-limits—just consider their higher fat content when making the rest of your meal.

EGGS

Consider them your pound-shedding partners in crime. Researchers from the University of Louisiana found that eating eggs for breakfast can cut your daily food intake by up to 415 calories. At less than 80 calories, a single egg is packed with fat-fighting vitamin D and high-quality proteins that keep you feeling full longer. And despite their bad press, if your cholesterol is healthy, you can eat eggs every day.

FISH

Low in calories, packed with protein, and a leading source of powerful omega-3s—seafood should top every grocery list. Yet women still don't get the recommended two servings a week. Why? Either they don't know how to cook seafood or they're concerned about things like mercury or chemical pollutants. If you're looking to add more seafood to your menu, salmon and scallops are good places to start. Salmon is well known for its hefty omega-3 content, which gives a rich, yet mild, flavor; it's also a great source of vitamin D, which is essential for strong bones and a healthy immune system. Just 3 ounces contain 52 percent of your recommended daily dose of niacin, a B vitamin that boosts energy and helps your body metabolize carbs and fat. (You'll get the most flavor from wild-caught species, such as Alaskan king.) And scallops are one of the leanest proteins around, with only 95 calories and less than 1 gram of fat per 3 ounces. (Bay scallops are soft, sweet, and more delicate-tasting, compared to steaklike sea scallops, but both are equally delicious and take just minutes to prepare.) Also, keep canned light tuna, chicken, and crabmeat in your pantry; they make it easy to quickly whip up high-protein snacks and meals in a pinch. (Make a big batch at the start of the week and use it to make sandwiches, add it on top of salads, or eat it with whole grain crackers as a satisfying midday snack.) You can find creative ways to make your classic tuna salad healthier and tastier on page 232.

YOGURT

It's no surprise that yogurt was one of the top foods associated with weight loss, according to a 20-year study by the Harvard T. H. Chan School of Public Health: It's packed with protein and calcium, and the Greek variety has even more—plus, its thick texture is traditionally achieved by straining, which removes not only the liquid whey, but also some of the sugar and salt. Recent research uncovered another benefit of consuming yogurt: Eating about 6 ounces of the low-fat variety three times a week was linked to a 31 percent lower risk of high blood pressure. However, some companies use thickeners to give yogurt that smooth consistency, so check the ingredients panel for milk protein concentrate or cornstarch, two common thickeners, and other unfamiliar ingredients. Something else to look for on the label: *lactobacillus.* In a study, participants who ate yogurt containing healthy bacteria called probiotics daily lost 3 to 4 percent of their body fat over 6 weeks, reports the *Journal of Functional Foods.* (The shift in gut bacteria prompted by probiotics may favor fat burning over fat storage, say study authors.)

WHEY

Research found that people who ate this protein (found in dairy foods and supplements) in place of other calories shed weight. It may also increase muscle, scientists say. A few sources: whey protein powder (about 24 grams per scoop), yogurt (5 grams per ½ cup), and milk (8 grams per 8 ounces).

GRAINS AND LEGUMES

Notice I'm not even uttering the "C" word here. That's because over the years, "carbohydrate" has become some kind of dieting curse word; use it, and people will flip out about how if you want to lose weight you need to lay off anything containing the stuff. But here's the thing: Remember, this isn't a diet plan. This isn't meant to teach you how to lose 10 pounds by tomorrow; it's meant to help you find a way of eating that feels satisfying, not depriving. It's meant to help you find something that will work over the long term. And when you're looking at your diet from that perspective, your body needs the fuel and energy that it gets from carbs. The key is focusing on the quality of the source and watching the quantity (forgo both, and you may start finding weight loss—or even weight maintenance—more challenging). Rather than another failed attempt at "giving up all carbs," try a more feasible approach: Swap processed carbs for unprocessed whole grains and beans like the following group.

QUINOA

This grain is loaded with protein, but unlike the protein in wheat, quinoa contains every amino acid needed for proper nutrition. With 5 grams of fiber per serving, it's the ultimate nutritious meal base. It cooks like rice and makes an excellent substitute for more common grains: Try using it as a bed for grilled chicken or fish, tossing it with roasted vegetables for a simple salad, or stirring in raisins, brown sugar, and milk for breakfast. (While quinoa may come out on top, you can also use brown rice and whole grain couscous as comparable alternatives.)

OATMEAL

The collective efforts of beta-glucan, a powerful class of fibers, and avenanthramides, which are unique to oats and have antioxidant properties, fuel the cereal grain's winning battle against LDL cholesterol. And get this: A study of satiety published in the *New England Journal of Medicine* showed that oatmeal more than doubled the stomach-filling potential of white bread. However, oatmeal's heart-smart, waistline-trimming reputation is so solid that you might not think to check the label. But some brands cram in artificial ingredients and sweeteners that displace the benefits. A better solution: Ditch the packets and stick with plain oats, then boost the flavor and nutrition of your morning meal with the quick recipes on page 230.

BEANS

Black beans, cannellini beans, pinto beans, chickpeas, lentils—because they serve up filling fiber and protein in addition to slow-digesting carbohydrates, beans and other legumes help keep you feeling fuller, longer. In fact, people who eat ³⁄₄ cup of beans per day have lower blood pressure and smaller waist sizes compared to those who don't eat beans. Beans are also packed with vitamins and minerals: Black beans, for example, are rich in magnesium; black-eyed peas are an excellent source of folate; and kidney beans pack iron, omega-3 fatty acids, and cancer-fighting antioxidants.

FRUITS AND VEGGIES

Regardless of your outlook, you'll be hard pressed to find a dietary lifestyle that doesn't advocate eating more vegetables. Many studies prove that a diet rich in fruits and veggies slows the absorption of sugar into your blood-stream, lowering your risk of diabetes. Plus, a veggie-and-fruit–rich diet prevents fatty substances from sticking to blood vessel walls, helping defend against heart disease. And the fiber in vegetables helps reduce blood choles-terol levels, while also helping you feel fuller on fewer calories. This is one instance where you can't get too much of a good thing. Here's a short list of the top picks.

LEAFY GREENS

Intentionally vague here. That's because we don't need to get into a debate over whether kale is king or spinach is the best. At the end of the day, leafy green vegetables all get top marks for being low in calories and fat and high in dietary fiber, vitamin C, folate, manganese, and vitamin K. Spinach, kale, arugula, broccoli, Brussels sprouts, chard, collard greens, red and green leaf lettuce, and cabbage are all good choices.

ROOT VEGETABLES

Think veggies that grow in the ground—carrots, sweet potatoes, turnips, pars-nips, beets. While they tend to contain more complex carbs than leafy greens do, they're also some of the very best sources of carotenoid antioxidants and vitamins A and C. And research has found that higher root vegetable intake is associated with a reduced risk for diabetes. (And, for the purposes of our big-picture thinking, let's go ahead and include "fruit" veggies in this group, as well. We're talking peppers, tomatoes, butternut squash—delicious, nutrient-packed produce picks that are technically labeled as fruits in botany circles, but which most of us consider to be veggies.)

MUSHROOMS

Okay, some will split hairs and call these fungi and not technically vegetables, but the USDA classifies them as veggies because they have so many of the nutritional attributes of vegetables. (You'll also find them in the produce section, so, yeah—let's call them vegetables.) Interesting bit about mushrooms: Research has found that they provide nutrients that bridge across core food groups—meaning stuff you'll find in produce, meats, and grains can also be found in 'shrooms. They are also a good source of niacin, selenium, and copper and an excellent source of riboflavin. Additionally, they contain potassium, dietary fiber, vitamin D, and calcium, four nutrients Americans should be consuming more of, according to the Dietary Guidelines for America.

RASPBERRIES

All berries, including blueberries, strawberries, raspberries, and blackberries, are rich in vitamin C, which has been shown to help combat stress. While all berries are great sources of hunger-quelling fiber, raspberries have the most. (One cup contains more fiber than four slices of whole grain bread and twice as much as 1 cup of blueberries.)

GRAPEFRUIT

In a study published in the *Journal of Medicinal Food,* obese adults who ate half a grapefruit before each of their three daily meals lost 3 more pounds over the course of 12 weeks than those who skipped the grapefruit appetizer.

APPLES

An apple a day may keep the extra pounds away! A study in the journal *Appetite* found that people who ate an apple consumed 15 percent fewer calories afterward than those who didn't eat the fruit. The fiber in apples slows digestion, and a medium apple has 4 filling grams of it. (Most of it's in the skin, so don't peel it!)

BANANAS

Research reveals that the yellow guys contain "resistant starch," a type of fiber that your body digests more slowly, which keeps your blood sugar levels stable and leaves you feeling satisfied for longer.

SIMPLE PANTRY STAPLES

Cooking healthy meals at home is easy when your pantry is stocked with some healthy staples. Here are a few essentials that can help you bring healthy ingredients together to make delicious meals with little to no planning. They're basic ingredients with long shelf lives, and they can be combined with other ingredients in countless ways.

OLIVE OIL

Dairy gets all the credit for fortifying your frame, but there may be another food that can help you bone up: olive oil. In a study published in the *Journal of Clinical Endocrinology and Metabolism,* people who consumed a Mediterranean diet plus virgin olive oil for 2 years saw an increase in osteocalcin, a protein that's a marker of bone growth. Those who didn't increase their oil intake experienced no such bone boon. To safeguard your skeleton and keep you feeling satiated longer after meals, drizzle it on roasted veggies and use it in homemade dressings.

CANNED, WHOLE, PEELED TOMATOES

The little-known secret behind most great Italian restaurants' red sauce is that it's made with canned tomatoes. That's because canned tomatoes are picked at the height of tomato season and canned immediately, preserving the intensely sweet, acidic flavor of summer tomatoes. Use them as the base for homemade salsa; combine with nothing more than olive oil and salt for a perfect pizza sauce; use as the base for a slow-cooked dish, such as baked chicken breasts; or make the perfect pasta sauce by simmering with onions, garlic, and red-pepper flakes.

CHICKEN STOCK

Restaurants typically use butter and cream as the base for most of their sauces, which explains why restaurant food can be so disastrous to your waistline. Using chicken stock—to moisten stuffing, build sauces, or braise meat and vegetables—gives you the flavors of roasted chicken and root vegetables with minimal caloric impact (about 10 calories per $\frac{1}{2}$ cup). Vegetable and beef stock are great options, as well. Combine the stock with equal parts red or white wine, plus shallots and herbs, and boil until it's reduced to sauce consistency (perfect for steak or chicken); stretch a pasta sauce without boosting calories by adding a few splashes of stock; or deglaze a skillet or a roasting pan you cooked meat in with a cup of stock, then add a few pinches of flour and a pat of butter for instant gravy.

BALSAMIC VINEGAR

Probably the most famous vinegar of all, beloved for its tangy-sweet taste. It's perfect as a base for building salad dressings and marinades, as well as a special secret touch when caramelizing onions, braising meat in a slow cooker, or quick-pickling vegetables. Combine with equal parts soy sauce, plus chopped garlic, for a great steak or chicken marinade; mix with two parts olive oil, a small spoonful of Dijon mustard, and salt and pepper for an all-purpose vinaigrette; cover onions or cucumbers with balsamic for 10 minutes for an instant pickle; or toss with chopped strawberries and pour over vanilla ice cream. (Trust me!)

SPICES

Your spice rack might be your best partner in crime in the kitchen: Strong food aromas can help you eat 5 to 10 percent less of a meal, according to research published in the journal *Flavour*. Study authors explain that people

GO NUTS!

"Tree nuts"—a group that includes pistachios, almonds, hazelnuts, and pecans—could slash your obesity risk, according to a study in *PLOS ONE*. Tossing back 28 grams a week (about a handful total) was associated with 10 percent less obesity and 7 percent less metabolic syndrome. One explanation? The high fiber and protein content of nuts may keep you full and prevent you from overeating other high-calorie foods, say study authors. Other studies conducted by the National Institutes of Health found that the omega-3 fatty acids in walnuts keep the stress hormones cortisol and adrenaline in check. And yes, peanut butter is in, too: In fact, a study in the *British Journal of Nutrition* found that adding peanuts or peanut butter to your breakfast can help curb hunger throughout the day. The fat, protein, and fiber in peanuts work together to help control your appetite. (Just keep it capped at 2 tablespoons.)

may unconsciously take smaller bites to regulate the amount of flavor they experience. Keep these spice staples on hand to mix into everything from omelets and smoothies to soups and side dishes: chili powder, curry powder, dried oregano, dried rosemary, dried thyme, garlic powder, ground cinnamon, ground cumin, paprika, and red-pepper flakes. You can also use spices in place of a marinade to add flavor to meat dishes in minutes. Just mix the spices together to make a rub, pat it all over beef or chicken, and cook as instructed. The best part is, there's no hard-and-fast rule on the perfect rub—simply tweak and refine your own blends based on your personal preferences and what you have in the pantry. Or, use these three mixes as a starting point.

BEEF / salt and pepper, garlic salt, ground red pepper, ground cumin, pinch of ground cinnamon

CHICKEN / salt and pepper, ground cumin, chili powder, brown sugar

FISH / salt and pepper, smoked paprika, thyme

QUICK TIPS:
FOOD PREP

95 **Blend in bananas.** Bananas help lend a thicker, creamier consistency to a smoothie. At the start of each week, dice a bunch of bananas and place them in a resealable plastic bag in your freezer. Not only will this save you prep time in the mornings, but it also means you won't have to add as much ice.

96 **Cut creatively.** Avoid messy stains and get at a pomegranate's arils faster by slicing it in half, then submerging it in a bowl of water. The seeds will sink while the pith floats, making them easy to separate.

97 **Seal in flavor.** Mix marinade ingredients well in a resealable plastic bag, drop in the meat, seal, shake, and refrigerate.

98 **Marinate in minutes.** When grilling flank or skirt steak, marinate it for 10 minutes after cooking, instead of before. It adds amazing, full flavor in a tenth of the time.

99 **Don't waste a drop of jam.** Don't throw out those last drips of jam in the jar; shake up a fruity vinaigrette, instead. Add equal parts oil and vinegar to the jar, give it a good shake, and season with salt and pepper to taste. (Find more easy vinaigrette recipes on pages 233 to 234.)

100 **Keep herbs fresher, longer.** Store fresh herbs as you would fresh flowers: in a jar of water on your countertop. Pluck off what you need, change the water daily, and they'll last two to three times longer than they would in the fridge. You'll get the most extra mileage from flat-leaf parsley.

101 **Crack eggs carefully.** Always crack an egg on a flat surface, never the edge of a bowl. Otherwise you'll risk eating shell shards and possibly contaminating your food.

102 **Eat leftovers for lunch.** A good soup is made a day in advance. Let it sit in the fridge overnight, then warm it gently and all the flavors will marry beautifully.

103 **Freeze in freshness.** Freeze fresh ginger and grate as needed. It will stay fresh for months.

104 **Simplify your shredding.** Spritz your cheese grater with non-stick spray before using it to make shredding—and cleaning—easier.

105 **Annotate your recipes.** If you change something and it works, write it down.

106 **Slice right.** The way you chop something has a major impact on the way it tastes. Zucchini takes on a spaghetti-like flavor when cut into wide, thin ribbons with a mandoline or sharp knife. Radishes sliced into matchsticks can add a peppery zing to dishes without overpowering other ingredients. Finely minced red onion or garlic (use a paring knife) has less of a bite than larger pieces. And a box grater can mellow out almost any veggie; use one to make produce "confetti" that can add delicate flavor and extra nutrition to your meal.

DO SOMETHING TODAY YOUR FUTURE SELF WILL THANK YOU FOR.

FITNESS FIX

13/

Quick & Easy Recipe Ideas

HOPEFULLY BY NOW YOU'RE starting to believe that eating in is not as time-consuming or difficult as you might have thought. Simple, cheap, fast, and delicious? Yep, it's possible. And you don't have to do some grand, unmanageable overhaul of your eating habits, either. Your goal: Make just *one* meal better today. Or make a few smart swaps throughout the day—replacing a slice of cheese with an extra handful of spinach to cut 100 calories from your omelet, or cutting about 77 calories per ounce by dressing your salad with lemon juice rather than balsamic vinaigrette.

In this chapter, you won't find set-in-stone meal plans or elaborate recipes with calorie counts and perfectly portioned serving sizes. Instead, you'll find approachable, affordable ingredients combined in a straightforward, easy-to-follow way. Why? Well, for starters, I think a lot of women get caught up in the numbers. They obsess over calories. I'm not going to say that it can't be helpful to count every calorie and log every bite of food—certainly, in some situations, these can can be useful tools for jump-starting weight loss and keeping healthy habits on track. But notice, I said *jump-start*. You won't find many slim-for-life people who count every single calorie and track every bite over the long term. It's just not sustainable; in fact, it's exhausting.

Remember, this isn't some 30-day challenge guaranteed to help you lose those last 10 pounds. Everything in this book can help you do that, of course, but it's not the main goal. This chapter is meant to be a tool to help you develop and strengthen your own, personal, healthy eating lifestyle—for the rest of your life. And to do that, it needs to fit with your lifestyle—now, and as it changes. So if you're a single woman cooking for one, these recipes will work for you. If you're a mom of five cooking for an entire family, these recipes will also work for you. Simply adjust the ingredient portions to match the number of portions you need. The same goes for your goals. If you're currently training for a marathon, you'll need an extra serving or two of healthy carbs each day to help keep you running strong and to keep your energy up; on the other hand, if you're trying to lose a few pounds before vacation, you might find it helpful to swap in some extra protein instead of the grains.

The point is, it doesn't matter where you're at now or where you're hoping to go—the ideas in this chapter can help you get there. Use these healthy recipes as a jumping-off point to help you think ahead about what you want to make each week—then tweak the ingredients based on what you like, what you have on hand, and what sounds good *to you*.

ALL-DAY EGGS

At 6 grams of protein each, eggs are hands-down one of the easiest, most affordable protein sources—serving up plenty of fat-fighting vitamin D, riboflavin, and vitamin B_{12} with every bite. When you're trying to eat healthy, eggs are an easy option for breakfast, lunch, dinner, or just as a snack. And because eggs will keep in your refrigerator for 3 to 5 weeks, you don't have to worry about pounding through a dozen in a week, either.

SWEET AND SAVORY SCRAMBLE / In a large nonstick skillet over medium heat, sauté spiralized sweet potato until it's soft and lightly browned; season with chili powder and a dash of salt and pepper. Add beaten eggs and scramble until the eggs are nearly set, then stir in shaved Parmesan.

DENVER SCRAMBLE / In a large nonstick skillet over medium heat, sauté chunks of ham with sliced mushrooms, onions, and bell peppers until the vegetables are soft and lightly browned. Add beaten eggs and scramble until the eggs are nearly set, then stir in a handful of sharp Cheddar.

CHILE SCRAMBLE / In a large nonstick skillet over low heat, scramble eggs gently. Stir in pieces of broken tortillas, canned roasted chiles, and diced tomatoes. Season with salt, pepper, and hot sauce.

SUNNY-SIDE UP ASPARAGUS / Roast or blanch asparagus spears until tender. Arrange four or five on a plate, top with sunny-side up eggs, and finish with a grating of Parmesan, salt, and pepper.

SIMPLE SHAKSHUKA / Preheat the oven to 400°F. Spoon jarred tomato sauce into ramekins or individual baking dishes. Crack an egg or two directly into the sauce, top with red-pepper flakes, and bake for about 10 minutes, until the egg whites just set.

RICOTTA AND CHIVE SCRAMBLE / In a nonstick pan over medium-low heat, heat a tablespoon of butter until brown, then add in beaten eggs. Slowly scramble until the eggs are soft and beginning to set, then fold in a few spoonfuls of ricotta cheese and freshly chopped chives. Serve on top of crusty bread.

SIMPLE EGG SALAD / In a medium bowl, combine chopped-up hard-boiled eggs with light mayo, Dijon mustard, capers, minced onion, and any fresh herbs you may have. Serve on a salad, in a pita, or as filling in a toasted English muffin.

BREAKFAST TACOS / In a large nonstick skillet over medium heat, scramble eggs with chopped scallions and hunks of cooked chicken sausage. Serve in warm tortillas topped with black beans, sliced avocado, and salsa.

EGG AND PESTO MELT / Spread toasted English muffins with a spoonful of pesto. Top with scrambled eggs and shredded mozzarella cheese. Place under the broiler until the cheese melts and bubbles.

MEXICAN BAKED EGGS / In a small saucepan over low-medium heat, simmer half a can of black beans with 1 cup of chicken stock. Crack two eggs directly into the mixture and cook until the whites are set. Top with plenty of hot sauce.

OATMEAL 2.0

Oatmeal is a quick and easy whole grain option you're probably used to reaching for in the morning, but if all you've ever done with it is sprinkle on some blueberrries or drizzle it with a little syrup, it's time to step things up. These combinations are anything but basic.

OATY EGG FLORENTINE / In a small bowl, combine $1/4$ cup chopped baby spinach and $1/2$ cup oatmeal. Top with 1 thin slice of Swiss cheese and 1 large egg, sunny-side up.

STRAWBERRIES AND CREAM / In a medium bowl, combine $1/4$ cup plain nonfat Greek yogurt, 1 table-spoon honey, $1/4$ cup sliced straw-berries, and $1/2$ cup oatmeal. Stir well and garnish with strawberry halves.

MAPLE-BACON OATMEAL / In a small skillet over medium heat, cook 2 slices of turkey bacon. In a small bowl, combine $1/2$ cup oatmeal with 2 tablespoons maple syrup, then crumble the bacon on top.

CHAI OATMEAL / In a small bowl, mix $1/2$ cup oatmeal with a pinch each of ground cardamom, cinnamon, cloves, and ginger, and $1/4$ cup low-fat milk. Drizzle with 1 teaspoon honey and 2 tablespoons slivered almonds.

CACIO E PEPE / Mix $1/2$ cup oatmeal with 2 tablespoons shredded pecorino Romano cheese and $1/2$ teaspoon freshly ground black pepper. Top with 2 teaspoons heart-healthy extra-virgin olive oil.

OVERNIGHT OATS / In a jar, combine $1/2$ cup oats, 1 cup unsweetened almond milk, and 1 teaspoon honey. Cover and refrigerate overnight. Top with two sliced strawberries and $1/2$ tablespoon almond slivers just before serving.

POWER SMOOTHIES

If only every meal could be as simple as the click of a button. Power through your morning or afternoon with one of these nutrient-dense smoothies.

MAKE A BETTER SMOOTHIE

Three simple tips for a richer, more nutritious blend every time.

» **WATCH YOUR CONSISTENCY** / For every 3 cups of produce, you'll need about 1 cup of liquid. Ice adds thickness, but too much of it can dilute the flavor and water down your smoothie. Boost consistency with ingredients like avocado, low-fat Greek yogurt, frozen bananas, canned pumpkin, and fruit. (Keep in mind that frozen fruit adds more texture than fresh. Bonus: It's less expensive, too.)

» **FILL UP FASTER** / Toss in hunger-squashing ingredients like wheat germ, ground flaxseed, and high-fiber fruits (think raspberries, blackberries, and avocados). Leave the peel on thin-skinned fruits such as pears and peaches. Add protein with a scoop of whey protein powder, tofu, cottage cheese, or peanut butter.

» **GO GREEN** / Kale, spinach, arugula, celery, fresh herbs (such as mint, parsley, and cilantro)—there are few greens that you can't toss into your blender. (Okay, maybe broccoli. It's healthy and delicious in so many ways, but it's not as smoothie-friendly.) If you find it hard to get your daily serving of greens, consider adding them to your smoothie. A handful of spinach might change the color, but it really won't alter the taste; however, sometimes veggies can be bitter, so shoot for a 70:30 fruit-to-greens ratio.

CAFFEINATED BANANA / Blend together 1 very ripe banana, ½ cup strong coffee, ½ cup 2% milk, 2 tablespoons peanut butter, 1 tablespoon agave syrup or honey, and 2 cups ice.

VITAMIN C MONSTER / Blend together 1 cup yogurt, ½ cup frozen papaya chunks, ½ cup frozen mango chunks, ½ cup frozen pineapple chunks, 1 cup orange juice, and 1 cup ice.

BRAIN BOOSTER / Blend together 1 cup pomegranate juice, 1 cup frozen blueberries, 1 cup yogurt, fresh basil to taste, and 1 tablespoon flax seeds.

EYE OPENER / Blend together 1 cup frozen chopped kale, 1 apple, 1 cup yogurt, fresh ginger as desired, and 1 cup ice.

AFTERNOON DELIGHT / Blend together 1 scoop chocolate protein powder, 1 tablespoon peanut butter, ½ cup chocolate milk, ½ cup spinach, and 2 cups ice.

SUPER SALADS

They're arguably the most utilized "diet" meals, but salads present two problems: Women either use the same boring, super-light ingredients (so they don't feel satisfied by what they've eaten) or they load up their lettuce with so many calorie-laden toppings that it hardly deserves to be categorized as a salad. Here, a few ways to slim down your salad.

LIGHTER DELI STYLE

Chicken, egg, tuna—they're inexpensive staples, but for all their protein-loaded, metabolism-boosting potential, when combined into a "salad," they are not often thought of as weight-loss allies (thanks to the massive amount of mayo used). But with a few simple tweaks, you can recreate the old standby into an awesome go-to option. (Make a big batch at the start of the week to save on prep time.) First, you want just enough binder (think: mayo) to lightly coat your ingredients. If you can't distinguish the individual ingredients in the salad, you've gone too far. Second, think about texture: Like a regular salad, protein-based salads benefit from crunch. Toasted nuts, celery, and apples are all excellent choices. Lastly, switch up what you pair the salad with. Have it over a bed of lettuce, on an open-faced English muffin, or with carrots or wheat crackers.

CURRIED CHICKEN DELI SALAD / Combine chicken, onion, carrot, golden raisins, mayo, and curry powder.

RIVIERA SALMON DELI SALAD / Combine salmon, olive oil, Dijon mustard, capers, and fresh parsley or dill.

TUSCAN TUNA DELI SALAD / Combine tuna, celery, olives, sundried tomatoes, olive oil, and lemon juice.

FIERY EGG SALAD / Combine hard-cooked eggs, onion, pickle, mayo, and sriracha or hot sauce.

FRESH MIXES

These flavor-packed combos are just as delicious as they are nutritious. Make them yourself or use them as a cheat sheet when you're ordering out.

APPLE-BLUE / Toss Bibb lettuce, red onion, apple, blue cheese, grilled chicken, and yogurt dressing.

MEDITERRANEAN / Toss arugula, tuna, hard-cooked egg, artichoke hearts, roasted peppers, olives, and balsamic vinegar.

ASIAN / Toss mixed greens, cucumber, mandarin oranges, chicken, almond slivers, and ginger-soy dressing.

CHOPPED / Toss iceberg, hard-cooked egg, ham, cherry tomatoes, carrots, red onion, and ranch dressing.

THAI / Toss buckwheat soba noodles, extra-firm tofu, carrots, red bell pepper, edamame, and sesame seeds.

SALMON / Toss Bibb lettuce, canned salmon, avocado, pink grapefruit, red onion, beets, and pistachios.

MOROCCAN / Toss arugula, chickpeas, avocado, yellow tomato, cucumber, red onion, golden raisins, and sunflower seeds.

SHRIMP / Toss romaine lettuce, shrimp, celery, red cabbage, grape tomatoes, and blue-cheese crumbles.

BERRY CHICKEN / Toss baby spinach, grilled chicken, strawberries, blueberries, yellow tomato, goat-cheese crumbles, and pecans.

DIY DRESSING

Considering how easy it is to make vinaigrette at home, it's hard to believe that people settle for store-bought dressings that are loaded with salt and high-fructose corn syrup. Here are five delicious homemade dressings to try. You can use a bowl and whisk, but a clean mason jar is even better. Add your base flavorings, then your vinegar and oil (no more than two parts oil to one part vinegar). Pour in the remaining seasonings and shake for 20 seconds. Store any leftovers in your fridge for up to a week.

THAI / Combine 1 tablespoon creamy peanut butter, 2 tablespoons rice wine vinegar, 2 tablespoons reduced-sodium soy sauce, 2 tablespoons fresh lime juice, and 1 teaspoon firmly packed brown sugar.

CHILI SPICE / Combine 1 tablespoon extra-virgin olive oil, 2 tablespoons fresh orange juice, 2 teaspoons white wine vinegar, $\frac{1}{2}$ teaspoon orange zest, $\frac{1}{2}$ teaspoon Dijon mustard, 1 large pinch kosher salt, and 1 large pinch chili powder.

MOROCCAN / Combine 1 tablespoon olive oil, $\frac{1}{2}$ teaspoon orange zest, 2 tablespoons lime juice, 1 tablespoon honey, 1 large pinch ground cinnamon, and $\frac{1}{4}$ teaspoon ground cumin.

BETTER BLUE CHEESE / Combine 1 teaspoon sugar, $1\frac{1}{2}$ teaspoons white wine vinegar, 2 tablespoons water, 2 tablespoons plain nonfat Greek yogurt, 2 tablespoons light canola mayonnaise, and 1 tablespoon blue-cheese crumbles.

BERRY VINAIGRETTE / Combine $\frac{1}{4}$ cup sliced strawberries, 1 tablespoon fresh orange juice, $1\frac{1}{2}$ teaspoons red wine vinegar, $\frac{1}{2}$ teaspoon orange zest, $\frac{1}{2}$ teaspoon sugar, 2 tablespoons plain nonfat Greek yogurt, and 1 large pinch kosher salt.

BETTER BURGERS

With minimal effort (and ingredients), you can whip up a protein-packed dinner in minutes. Shake up your standard burger with these mouthwatering, super-simple alternatives—each packed with lean protein and healthy fats to keep you totally satisfied.

SALMON BURGER / In a food processor, pulse 12 ounces of salmon fillet pieces for 1 minute. In a medium bowl, combine the salmon with 1 teaspoon finely chopped fresh rosemary, $\frac{1}{3}$ cup panko bread crumbs, 1 egg white, and 2 teaspoons lemon zest. Form into 4 patties. Grill over medium-high heat for 4 to 5 minutes, then flip and grill for another 4 to 5 minutes.

BUILD A BETTER SALAD

Follow these six simple rules to build a better salad every time.

GET CREATIVE WITH YOUR BASE /
A salad doesn't have to start with iceberg. Robust, dark greens add power nutrients such as folate and vitamins A, C, and K for negligible calories, while the fiber and complex carbs in whole grains fill you up. Try one of these: 1½ cups romaine, Bibb, frisée, spinach, or arugula (or any combination), plus ½ cup cooked grains, such as quinoa or whole grain couscous, or 1 to 2 ounces soba noodles or whole wheat linguine.

PUMP UP THE PROTEIN /
Protein provides the belly-filling satisfaction that transforms a side salad into a main dish. Get your dose from lean sources such as chicken, fish, beans, or tofu. Try one of these: 2 ounces fish (such as canned or fresh salmon; trout; or smoked blue fish); 5 large shrimp (broiled, boiled, or grilled); 2 ounces lump crabmeat; 3 ounces skinless chicken breast (broiled or grilled); ¼ to 1 cup cooked beans (such as chickpeas or black beans); or 2 ounces cooked tofu.

ADD COLOR /
Vibrant produce doesn't just make your salad look pretty—it also ensures that your dish is loaded with vitamins and other nutrients. Just one-quarter of a red bell pepper provides more than 40 percent of your daily vitamin A needs, while tomatoes are full of cancer-fighting lycopene. Try one (or more!) of these: ¼ cup chopped red, yellow, or orange bell pepper; ¼ to ½ cup chopped red, yellow, orange, or green tomato (about 1 medium); ¼ cup chopped red, golden, or Chioggia beet; ¼ cup shredded carrot; or 1 or 2 medium slices red onion.

TOSS IN SOMETHING SOFT /
A touch of softness gives a salad balance and texture and makes it extra satisfying. A soft cheese also provides calcium and protein, plus a hint of saltiness. Just be mindful of how much you toss in—cheese and other rich ingredients can ratchet up the calorie count. Try one of these: 1 to 2 teaspoons soft cheese, such as feta, goat, or blue cheese; ⅛ avocado; or 1 heart of palm.

FIRE UP THE FLAVOR /
Spicy, tart, or sweet ingredients add a layer of depth and complexity to a salad and can offset some of the more bitter greens and veggies. For example, fresh fruit will satisfy a sweet tooth, while zingy fresh herbs boost flavor but not fat. Try one of these: ½ cup citrus fruit, such as fresh orange, lime, or grapefruit; tangy veggies, such as radishes, scallions, chives, grated or pickled ginger, or jalapeño, to taste; or zesty herbs, such as cilantro, basil, oregano, or tarragon, to taste.

TOP IT OFF WITH SOME CRUNCH /
Crispy, crunchy ingredients wake up your palate and are the perfect contrast to soft greens, noodles, and grains. Try one of these: 1 to 2 teaspoons nuts, such as pecans, walnuts, peanuts, macadamia nuts, almonds, or pine nuts; 1 to 2 teaspoons seeds, such as pumpkin, sunflower, sesame, or poppy; or ⅛ cup whole grain croutons. (Make your own by toasting a whole wheat baguette or pita.)

TURKEY BURGER / In a medium bowl, combine 12 ounces ground turkey, 2 tablespoons Dijon mustard, 2 tablespoons finely minced shallot, and 2 tablespoons chopped fresh parsley. Form into 4 patties and grill over medium-high heat for 5 to 6 minutes, then flip and grill for another 5 to 6 minutes, or until the burgers reach an internal temperature of 165°F.

BLACK BEAN BURGER / In a food processor, combine $1^1/_2$ cups canned no-salt-added black beans (rinsed and drained); $^1/_2$ yellow bell pepper, sliced; $^1/_3$ cup roughly chopped red onion; $^3/_4$ cup shredded carrot; $^1/_3$ cup dry quick-cooking oats, $2^1/_2$ teaspoons canola oil, and $^1/_2$ teaspoon cumin. Pulse 2 to 3 minutes, or until combined. Form into 4 patties. Lightly coat a piece of foil with cooking spray and place the foil on the grill. Cook the patties on the foil over medium-high heat for 5 minutes, then flip and cook for 5 minutes more.

BISON BURGER / In a medium bowl, combine 12 ounces ground grass-fed bison, $^1/_2$ cup chopped onion, $^1/_2$ teaspoon garlic powder, and $^1/_4$ teaspoon smoked paprika. Form into 4 patties. Grill over medium-high heat for 5 to 6 minutes, then flip and grill for another 5 to 6 minutes, or until the burgers reach an internal temperature of 155°F.

TASTY CHICKEN COMBINATIONS

At 110 calories and an impressive 23 grams of protein, skinless, boneless chicken breast clocks in as one of the most revered fat-burning foods you can eat. But without the right prep work, chicken can be, well, pretty boring. Here you'll find four different prep methods and 35 different delicious combinations to take your weekly lunch and dinner staple to the next level.

STIR-FRY

Cut a raw chicken breast into bite-size pieces or thin strips. In a nonstick skillet over medium-high heat, cook the chicken for 3 to 5 minutes, until browned, and add one of the following groups of ingredients—in the order listed—and cook for 5 more minutes, stirring frequently, until chicken reaches an internal temperature of at least 165°F.

BELL PEPPER MIX / Add 1 tablespoon reduced-sodium soy sauce; 2 teaspoons sesame oil; $\frac{1}{2}$ cup green or red bell pepper strips; $\frac{1}{4}$ medium onion, cut lengthwise into strips; and $\frac{1}{2}$ teaspoon red-pepper flakes.

VEGGIE BLEND / Add 1 tablespoon hoisin sauce; 2 teaspoons sesame oil; $\frac{1}{3}$ cup matchstick carrots; $\frac{1}{3}$ cup chopped celery; 1 scallion, sliced; and 2 tablespoons chopped unsalted peanuts.

ASPARAGUS AND CASHEW / Add 1 tablespoon reduced-sodium soy sauce, 2 teaspoons sesame oil, $\frac{1}{2}$ cup asparagus tips, and 2 tablespoons chopped unsalted cashews.

SWEET LEMON / Add 1 tablespoon reduced-sodium soy sauce; 1 tablespoon lemon juice; 1 teaspoon lemon zest; 1 teaspoon honey; 1 clove garlic, crushed; $\frac{1}{2}$ cup snow peas; and 1 cup chopped celery.

ASIAN BROCCOLI / Add 1 egg, beaten; $\frac{1}{2}$ cup (or more) chopped broccoli; $\frac{1}{4}$ medium onion, cut lengthwise into long strips; $\frac{1}{2}$ teaspoon red-pepper flakes; and 1 tablespoon reduced-sodium soy sauce.

HOISIN SNOW PEAS / Add 1 egg, beaten; $\frac{1}{2}$ cup snow peas; $\frac{1}{2}$ cup green or red bell pepper strips; $\frac{1}{4}$ onion, cut lengthwise into long strips; and 1 tablespoon hoisin sauce.

BASIC BAKE

Preheat the oven to 350°F and douse your chicken in one of the sauces below. Bake uncovered for 20 to 25 minutes or until the chicken reaches an internal temperature of 165°F at its thickest part.

MELTED FIESTA / Combine 2 tablespoons jalapeño cheese dip, 2 tablespoons salsa, and 1 tablespoon water.

HONEY MUSTARD / Combine 2 tablespoons Dijon mustard, 2 tablespoons honey, and 1 teaspoon olive oil.

CREAM OF MUSHROOM / Combine 2 tablespoons condensed mushroom soup and 2 tablespoons water.

PESTO / Combine 2 tablespoons pesto and 2 tablespoons reduced-sodium chicken broth.

SWEET AND SOUR / Combine 2 tablespoons reduced-sodium soy sauce and 1/4 cup crushed pineapple with juice.

COCONUT CURRY / Combine 3 tablespoons chicken broth, 2 tablespoons light coconut milk, and 1/4 teaspoon curry powder.

APPLE GLAZE / Combine 1/3 cup chicken broth, 1 tablespoon maple syrup, and 1 tablespoon apple juice.

BBQ SAUCE / Combine 3 tablespoons red wine vinegar; 1 tablespoon barbecue sauce; and 1 clove garlic, crushed.

HOT STUFF / Combine 2 tablespoons hot sauce, 2 tablespoons Worcestershire sauce, and 1/4 teaspoon chili powder.

HERBED CITRUS / Combine 2 tablespoons lemon juice, 2 tablespoons orange marmalade, and 1/4 teaspoon rosemary.

STUFFED

Preheat the oven to 350°F. Pound your chicken breast so it's uniformly thin. (Use a meat tenderizer, or cover the chicken with plastic wrap and pound with a pan or the bottom of a glass.) Arrange the following ingredients on the breast, roll it up, and secure it with toothpicks or kitchen twine. Bake uncovered for 20 to 25 minutes, or until the chicken reaches an internal temperature of 165°F.

HAM AND CHEESE / 1 slice Cheddar cheese, 2 slices deli ham, and 1/4 teaspoon black pepper.

STROMBOLI / 1 slice mozzarella cheese; 3 slices pepperoni; and 3 leaves fresh basil, chopped.

PIZZA / 1 slice mozzarella; 1/4 cup chopped tomatoes; and 3 leaves fresh basil, chopped.

SPINACH STUFFED / 1 small handful baby spinach leaves, chopped; 1 tablespoon blue-cheese crumbles; and 1 clove garlic, crushed.

DELI STYLE / 1 slice mozzarella, 1 slice salami, and 1 tablespoon chopped roasted red pepper.

SUN-DRIED TOMATO / $1\frac{1}{2}$ tablespoons part-skim ricotta cheese, 1 tablespoon chopped sun-dried tomatoes, and $\frac{1}{4}$ teaspoon oregano.

MEDITERRANEAN / $1\frac{1}{2}$ tablespoons part-skim ricotta cheese, 1 tablespoon diced olives, and $\frac{1}{4}$ teaspoon lemon zest.

PARMESAN PESTO / 1 tablespoon pesto, 1 tablespoon shredded Parmesan cheese, and $\frac{1}{4}$ teaspoon black pepper.

GRILLED

Soak the chicken in these marinades for at least an hour. Heat a grill or place a nonstick skillet over medium-high heat on the stove. Cook for 3 to 5 minutes per side, or until the chicken reaches an internal temperature of 165°F at its thickest part.

RED WINE DRESSED / Combine 2 tablespoons red wine; 1 teaspoon barbecue sauce; and 1 clove garlic, crushed.

WHITE WINE DRESSED / Combine 2 tablespoons white wine; 1 clove garlic, crushed; and $\frac{1}{4}$ teaspoon thyme.

RICH AND CREAMY / Combine 2 tablespoons plain yogurt and $\frac{1}{4}$ teaspoon dill.

MARGARITAVILLE / Combine 2 tablespoons lime juice, 1 teaspoon olive oil, and $\frac{1}{4}$ teaspoon cilantro.

CUMIN AND LIME / Combine 2 tablespoons lime juice, $\frac{1}{4}$ teaspoon cumin, and $\frac{1}{4}$ teaspoon red-pepper flakes.

LEMON ZEST / Combine 2 tablespoons lemon juice, $\frac{1}{4}$ teaspoon lemon zest, and $\frac{1}{4}$ teaspoon black pepper.

BALSAMIC HERB / Combine 2 tablespoons vinaigrette and $\frac{1}{4}$ teaspoon rosemary.

GINGER SPICED / Combine 2 tablespoons orange juice, $\frac{1}{4}$ teaspoon powdered ginger, and $\frac{1}{4}$ teaspoon cilantro.

HEALTHIER CHICKEN FINGERS

Crispy chicken fingers are one of my favorite foods, but I know they're not one of the best options to have on the regular. When I'm craving a healthier alternative, I make crusted chicken at home. It's easy: Crack an egg into a shallow bowl, beat it, dip the chicken in it, and then roll the chicken in a plate of one of these coatings.

» **GO NUTS** / ⅓ cup finely chopped nuts

» **ITALIAN** / 1 tablespoon finely grated Parmesan cheese, 1 tablespoon Italian bread crumbs, and a pinch of black pepper

» **FAUX FRIED** / ½ cup crushed corn or bran flakes, or ½ cup panko bread crumbs

O-JUICED / Combine 2 tablespoons orange juice, 1 tablespoon hoisin sauce, and ¼ teaspoon red-pepper flakes.

RED-PEPPER POP / Combine 1 tablespoon reduced-sodium soy sauce, 1 teaspoon sesame oil, and ¼ teaspoon red-pepper flakes.

SLOW COOKER

Too busy to cook? Don't like cooking? Well, you don't have to slave over the stove for hours—just grab a slow cooker and try one of these simple, super-nutritious recipes that practically make themselves. Simply add the ingredients in the order listed—then enjoy the healthy leftovers for the rest of the week!

SLOW COOKER ITALIAN CHICKEN SOUP / In a slow cooker, combine 1 pound boneless, skinless chicken breasts, cut into cubes; 1 medium onion, 1 zucchini, and 1 red pepper, all diced; 15 ounces cannellini beans (drained and rinsed); 15 ounces diced tomatoes; 2 cups chopped frozen kale; and 6 cups low-sodium chicken broth. Season with 1 tablespoon dried basil, 1 tablespoon dried oregano, ½ tablespoon garlic powder, ½ teaspoon salt, and ½ teaspoon red-pepper flakes. Cook on low for 8 hours or high for 4 hours.

SLOW COOKER WHITE CHICKEN CHILI / In a slow cooker, place

1¼ pounds boneless, skinless chicken cut into cubes. Top with two 15-ounce cans great northern or navy beans and one 15-ounce can white corn. In a medium bowl, combine 1 envelope low-sodium taco seasoning, 1 can (4 ounces) chopped green chiles, ½ teaspoon cumin, 1 can (15 ounces) cream-style sweet corn, and 14 ounces chicken broth. Pour over the ingredients in the slow cooker. Cook on low for 8 to 10 hours.

SLOW COOKER BURRITO BOWLS / In a slow cooker, combine 1 diced onion, 1 diced bell pepper, 1¼ cups black beans, 1 cup uncooked brown rice, 1½ cups diced tomatoes, ½ cup water, 1 teaspoon paprika, and ½ teaspoon ground cumin. Cook on low for about 3 hours. Serve and top with grated cheese, avocado, or sour cream.

SLOW COOKER PORK RAGU / In a large skillet, heat a few teaspoons olive oil over medium-high heat. Season a 2½-pound boneless pork loin with ½ teaspoon salt and ¼ teaspoon each of pepper, rosemary, and thyme. Brown all sides of the pork in the skillet for 3 to 4 minutes per side. Coat the inside of a slow cooker with cooking spray, and place the pork inside; top with 1 can (28 ounces) crushed tomatoes, ¾ cup chicken stock, ½ cup chopped onion, ⅓ cup grated carrots, 1 tablespoon tomato paste, ½ teaspoon minced garlic, and a splash of red wine. Cook on low for 8 hours or high for 4 to 5 hours. Use two forks to roughly shred the pork into large pieces. Simmer for an additional 30 minutes, then serve over pasta or vegetable noodles.

PIZZA

If you speed-dial your local pizza spot once a week, you're not alone: About 18 percent of Americans dive into some slices at least that often. The problem: Revised USDA guidelines from a few years ago singled out pizza as the second-highest source of saturated fat and the third-highest source of sodium in the American diet. That doesn't mean you have to give up this tasty and inexpensive meal altogether. Make it at home and you can satisfy your craving while saving hundreds of calories per serving.

BARBECUE CHICKEN PIZZA / Preheat the oven to 500°F. Place two small thin prebaked pizza crusts (like Boboli) on a baking sheet or pizza stone. Spread each with a little more than $1/4$ cup barbecue sauce; $3/4$ cup shredded smoked gouda; $1/4$ cup red onion, thinly sliced; $1/2$ cup cooked chicken, cubed, sliced, or shredded; and a few thin slices of jalapeño as desired. Bake for about 8 minutes, until the crust is golden and the cheese is fully melted. Top with fresh cilantro.

ARUGULA, CHERRY TOMATO, AND PROSCIUTTO PIZZA / Preheat the oven to 500°F. Place one large prebaked crust (like Boboli) on a baking sheet or pizza stone. Cover with 1 cup pizza sauce, $1^{1}/_{2}$ cups shredded part-skim mozzarella, and 2 cups cherry tomatoes. Bake for about 8 minutes, until the crust is golden and the cheese is completely melted. Remove the crust to a cutting board and immediately top with 2 cups arugula, 6 slices of prosciutto (torn or cut into thin slices), and shaved or grated Parmesan cheese.

HAWAIIAN MINI PIZZAS / Preheat the oven to 425°F. Place 4 English muffin halves on a baking sheet, and spread each with about 1 tablespoon tomato sauce; top with $1/4$ cup shredded mozzarella cheese, 2 slices deli ham (cut into strips), pineapple chunks, and pickled jalapeños to taste. Bake for 15 to 20 minutes, until the cheese is melted and bubbling and the bottoms of the English muffins are slightly crisp.

PESTO-GOAT CHEESE MINI PIZZAS / Preheat the oven to 425°F. Place 4 English muffin halves on a baking sheet, and spread each with about $1/2$ tablespoon pesto; top each with 1 tablespoon goat cheese, chopped green or kalamata olives, red onion slices, and 1 quartered artichoke heart (bottled or canned). Bake for 15 to 20 minutes, until the cheese is melted and bubbling and the bottoms of the English muffins are slightly crisp.

SAUSAGE AND PEPPER MINI PIZZAS / Preheat the oven to 425°F. Place 4 English muffin halves on a baking sheet, and spread each with about 1 tablespoon tomato sauce. Top each with $1/4$ cup shredded mozzarella cheese, 3 slices cooked chicken sausage, and roasted red peppers as desired;

season to taste with red-pepper flakes. Bake for 15 to 20 minutes, until the cheese is melted and bubbling and the bottoms of the English muffins are slightly crisp. Garnish with fresh basil leaves.

SIMPLE SIDES & SMALL BITES

From sweet to savory, all of these recipes share one thing in common: They're healthy, quick options that you can enjoy as a side to your main meal—or as an easy snack throughout your day.

SWEET POTATO FRIES / Preheat the oven to 425°F. Peel and cut 2 medium sweet potatoes into 12 equal wedges. Place them on a large baking sheet and toss with $1/2$ tablespoon olive oil; season with salt, pepper, and ground red pepper to taste. Spread in an even layer and bake for about 18 to 24 minutes (or until lightly browned), turning occasionally.

HONEY ROASTED CARROTS / Preheat the oven to 400°F. Toss 8 medium-size peeled carrots with 1 tablespoon olive oil, 2 tablespoons honey, $1/2$ tablespoon thyme leaves, and a generous amount of salt and pepper. Spread in an even layer on a baking sheet and cook for about 35 minutes, until brown on the outside and tender all the way through.

GARLIC-LEMON SPINACH / In a large skillet or saucepan over medium-low heat, heat 1 tablespoon olive oil. Add 3 cloves garlic (thinly sliced) and a pinch of red-pepper flakes, and cook gently for about 3 minutes, until the garlic is lightly browned. Add a few handfuls of spinach and cook, moving the uncooked spinach to the bottom of the pan with tongs, for about 5 minutes, until fully wilted. Drain off any excess water from the bottom of the pan. Stir in the juice of 1 lemon and season to taste with salt and black pepper.

SAUTÉED BRUSSELS SPROUTS / In a large skillet, heat $1/4$ cup olive oil over medium-high heat. Add $1 1/2$ to 2 pounds halved Brussels sprouts, as desired. Season with salt and pepper, and cook until caramelized, stirring frequently (about 8 to 10 minutes). Add 1 cup peeled, cubed apple pieces, a few teaspoons chopped garlic, and a handful of pine nuts, as desired, then sauté for another few minutes.

PARMESAN ASPARAGUS / Preheat the oven to 400°F. Lightly coat the spears with olive oil, salt, pepper, and a good grating of Parmesan cheese. Lay them out on a baking sheet and roast for about 12 minutes, until the spears are tender and the cheese is lightly browned. Squeeze lemon over the top before serving.

SPICY CHICKPEAS / In a skillet over medium heat, sauté 2 cloves of minced garlic and a few pinches of red-pepper flakes in olive oil until fragrant. Stir in canned, drained chickpeas and cook until heated through.

KALE CHIPS / Preheat the oven to 325°F. Chop a bunch of dry kale leaves (dinosaur kale, curly kale, or a mixture), drizzle with olive oil, and sprinkle with your choice of seasoning blends: lemon zest and sea salt; paprika, chipotle pepper, and sea salt; roasted sesame oil, roasted sesame seeds, and sea salt;

or shredded white Cheddar cheese and freshly ground black pepper. Toss and place on a baking sheet. Bake for 20 to 35 minutes, or until crispy.

ROSEMARY PARMESAN POPCORN / In a small bowl, drizzle 3 cups popped popcorn with 1 teaspoon olive oil. Sprinkle with 1 teaspoon finely chopped fresh rosemary and 1 tablespoon grated Parmesan cheese, then toss well to coat evenly. Top with black pepper.

PIÑA COLADA POPCORN / In a small skillet over low heat, melt 1 teaspoon extra-virgin coconut oil for about 15 seconds, or microwave it on High in a small glass dish for 30 seconds. In a small bowl, drizzle 3 cups popped popcorn with the oil. Sprinkle with 1 finely chopped ring of dried pineapple, 2 teaspoons sweetened coconut flakes, and $\frac{1}{8}$ teaspoon salt, then toss well to coat evenly.

CURRY CHIPOTLE POPCORN / In a small skillet over low heat, heat $1\frac{1}{2}$ teaspoons canola oil, $\frac{1}{2}$ teaspoon curry powder, $\frac{1}{4}$ teaspoon ground chipotle or chili powder, and $\frac{1}{8}$ teaspoon salt. Whisk gently for 1 to 2 minutes, until the oil begins to bubble. In a small bowl, drizzle 3 cups popped popcorn with the curry mixture, then toss well to coat evenly.

LEMON DILL POPCORN / In a small bowl, drizzle 3 cups popped popcorn with 1 teaspoon olive oil. Sprinkle with 1 teaspoon oregano, $\frac{1}{2}$ teaspoon dill, $\frac{1}{2}$ teaspoon lemon zest, and $\frac{1}{8}$ teaspoon salt, then toss well to coat.

SUGAR 'N' SPICE POPCORN / In a small bowl, drizzle 3 cups popped popcorn with 1 teaspoon flaxseed oil. Sprinkle with 1 teaspoon powdered sugar, $\frac{1}{2}$ teaspoon ground cinnamon, $\frac{1}{4}$ teaspoon ground nutmeg, and $\frac{1}{8}$ teaspoon salt, then toss well to coat evenly.

CRAN-CHOCOLATE POPCORN / In a small glass bowl, microwave 1 tablespoon dark chocolate chips for about 45 seconds, until they're just beginning to melt. Mix well with a rubber spatula until the chocolate is about three-quarters of the way melted; some lumps should remain. Put 3 cups popped popcorn into a medium bowl and top with the melted chocolate. Sprinkle with 2 tablespoons dried cranberries and $\frac{1}{8}$ teaspoon salt, then mix thoroughly. Place in the refrigerator for 10 minutes to harden the chocolate.

PEANUT BUTTER PROTEIN BALLS / In a medium bowl, mix 2 cups peanut butter, 2 scoops chocolate whey protein powder, $\frac{1}{4}$ cup molasses, 2 tablespoons honey, and 2 tablespoons whole flaxseeds. Form into walnut-size balls. Place on a baking sheet and freeze for 2 hours.

SKINNY SAUCES & DIPS

Healthy cooking doesn't have to be bland and boring. Utilizing simple sauces and dips can amp up the flavor of a dish—and, if made right, they can do it without adding unwanted calories. All of these make 1 to 2 cups and will keep fresh in the fridge for about a week. (The pesto and roasted garlic will last for up to 2.) Try using them to top off fresh meat dishes, as spreads on sandwiches, or as simple sides with a serving of vegetatables.

PESTO / In a food processor, combine 2 cloves garlic (chopped), 2 tablespoons pine nuts, 3 cups fresh basil leaves, and ¼ cup Parmesan, plus a few pinches of salt and pepper. Pulse until the basil is chopped. With the motor running, slowly drizzle a few teaspoons olive oil until fully incorporated and a paste forms. To keep it extra fresh and green, float a thin layer of oil on top before storing.

GUACAMOLE / Finely mince two cloves peeled garlic, then apply a pinch of salt and use the side of your knife to work the garlic into a paste. Scoop the garlic into a bowl, then add ¼ cup minced red onion, 1 tablespoon minced jalapeño, and 2 ripe avocados (peeled and pitted); mash until the avocados are pureed but still slightly chunky. Stir in the juice of 1 lemon or lime, chopped cilantro (if using), and salt to taste. Guacamole will keep for 4 to 6 days in the refrigerator.

ROASTED GARLIC / Preheat the oven to 325°F. Separate one head of garlic into cloves and peel them; place in the center of a large piece of aluminum foil and drizzle with 1 tablespoon olive oil. Place on a baking sheet and bake for 35 to 40 minutes, until the garlic is soft enough to spread like warm butter.

ROMESCO / In a medium skillet over medium heat, heat 1 tablespoon olive oil. Add 2 slices bread, torn into small pieces; 2 tablespoons chopped almonds; 2 cloves chopped garlic; and 1 teaspoon smoked paprika. Sauté for about 5 minutes, until the bread is lightly golden and crunchy. Transfer to a blender and add 2 tablespoons olive oil, 6 ounces roasted red peppers, 1 tablespoon red wine vinegar, and a pinch of salt and pepper. Puree until smooth.

CHIMICHURRI / In a food processor, combine 1 cup roughly chopped parsley, 1 clove garlic, ½ teaspoon salt, 2 tablespoons water, 1½ tablespoons red wine vinegar, ¼ cup oil, ½ teaspoon sugar, and 1 tablespoon minced jalapeño. Pulse until fully blended.

ONE-STEP HUMMUS / In a food processor, combine 1 clove garlic (chopped), 1 can (15 ounces) chickpeas (drained and rinsed), 2 tablespoons tahini, 2 tablespoons lemon juice, 2 tablespoons extra-virgin olive oil, 2 tablespoons water, ½ teaspoon ground cumin, and ½ teaspoon salt; blend until smooth.

DIPPING PARTNERS

Give the pita chips a break—try one of these low-cal swaps, instead.

» **ENDIVE** / Put a dab of dip in the center of a boat-shaped leaf and roll it up.

» **OKRA** / Season with olive oil, salt, and pepper, then roast at 400°F for 20 minutes.

» **SWEET POTATOES** / Cut into wedges and give them the same treatment as okra.

» **SHRIMP** / Boil with a little crab boil seasoning and lemon juice.

» **SUMMER SQUASH** / Slice into rounds or matchsticks, then dust lightly with salt.

» **SUGAR SNAP PEAS** / Eat them raw. They're crunchy, low-cal (just 14 calories per 10 pods), and full of vitamin C.

QUICK TIPS: COOKING

107 **Add dried fruit to oatmeal.** Pop it in before you add the milk or water. The fruit will cook and plump up slightly, adding a juicier, more intense taste.

108 **Salt it, then chill it.** When making a whole roast chicken, salt it, then chill it, uncovered, in the fridge for the day. This helps season the bird and dries out the skin so it crisps perfectly when cooked. Remove it from the fridge an hour before you plan to put it in the oven, and add herbs and aromatics like garlic or shallots.

109 **Is the meat done yet? The answer's in the palm of your hands.** Hold your hand in front of you, palm up. Keeping your hand relaxed, touch your thumb and index finger together. Now, press the fleshy area under your thumb with a finger from your other hand. That's what rare feels like. Now, press your thumb and middle finger together—the fleshy area under your thumb now feels like medium cooked meat. Repeat with your ring finger for medium-well and your pinky for well-done. Now that you know what it should feel like, press the top of the meat (quickly!) with your finger as it's cooking. This trick works for boneless chicken (always cook well-done) and red-meat steaks and chops (like pork and lamb).

110 **Rescue overcooked meat.** Slice it thinly, put it on a plate, and top it with chopped tomato, onion, and jalapeño. Add olive oil and fresh lime juice (or a few spoonfuls of vinaigrette). The acid and the oil will restore much-needed moisture and fat to the meat.

111 **Get the juiciest citrus.** Zap lemons, limes, or oranges for 15 seconds in the microwave before squeezing them. The fruit will yield twice as much juice.

112 **Use up those left-overs.** Use eggs to quickly transform leftovers—vegetables, a hunk of cheese, the last few slices of bread—into a savory frittata. (Just make sure egg-based dishes, such as casseroles and quiches, are cooked to an internal temperature of 160°F or higher by using a food thermometer.)

113 **Double-dip.** Cooking some pasta? Blanch a few handfuls of spring veggies at the same time, in the very same pot. Broccoli and French green beans, for instance, are perfect partners for penne. Just toss 'em into the boiling water with a few minutes to go, drain everything together in a big colander, add a little marinara sauce, and voilà—dinner is done and you have one less dish to wash. Score!

114 **Add an egg.** A runny-yolked fried egg adds instant richness (not to mention healthy fat and pro-tein) to pasta, rice and grain dishes—even pizza. Seriously: When in doubt, throw an egg on top of it.

115 **Smooth your shell-fish.** Before cooking mussels or clams, soak them in water with a few table-spoons of flour for 30 min-utes. As they open to ingest the flour, they'll expel any sand or grit they contain.

LIFE IS SHORT. EAT YOUR VEGGIES. DRINK YOUR WATER. BUT ENJOY THE CUPCAKE.

FITNESS FIX

PART III

KEEP IT
GOING

14 /

A Stronger Body— No Sweat!

WHILE THE MAJORITY OF this book focuses on better eating and exercise habits, there's another piece of the puzzle you're likely neglecting: To speed your results, research shows that what you do when you're not exercising is nearly as important as (if not more important than) the workout itself.

Before you roll your eyes and think, "Oh, great, one more thing to add to my already maxed out to-do list," hear me out. Exercise is literally a process of breaking down your muscle fibers, creating tiny microscopic tears; as soon as you slip off your sneakers after a workout, your body starts repairing that "damage" to your muscles. In fact, it's this recovery process—not the actual workout itself—that makes you stronger and leaner.

But it goes far beyond just crashing on the couch after a tough workout. Overlook the minimum-effort moves in this chapter and you could be stalling your progress. Follow these five secrets to use your downtime to increase energy, boost metabolism, reduce soreness, and drop weight faster.

SNEAK IN MORE SHUT-EYE

I know, I know—if you dropped a pound every time you heard about the advantages of sleep, you'd never have to work out again. I truly realize and value its importance, and yet I'm still guilty of logging way too many nights at far fewer than the standard 8-hour recommendation. But even if you think you operate just fine on less-than-average hours (like I do), prioritizing shut-eye truly may be one of the best things you can do to meet your body-shaping goals.

For starters, sleep increases production of tissue-repairing growth hormones, meaning you'll score some of your best muscle recovery under the covers. When Stanford University researchers had 1,000 volunteers report the number of hours they slept each night, they found the participants who got fewer than 8 hours of sleep per night had a higher body fat content. It's a weight-gain double whammy: Lack of sleep prompts your body to consume more calories and shuts down its ability to recognize a full stomach. When you're tired, your gut produces more ghrelin, a chemical that triggers sugar cravings. Meanwhile, fatigue suppresses leptin, a fat-cell hormone that tells your brain, "Okay, stop eating now." Then, there's the possibly larger issue: When you're awake more hours of the day, you have more opportunities to eat.

Your sweet spot: somewhere between 6 and 8 hours a night. A study found that people who snoozed for fewer than 6 were more likely to suffer a stroke or heart attack, and those who got more than 8 were also more likely to have heart woes. Too little sleep is associated with higher levels of stress hormones, while too much time between the sheets may indicate an underlying condition like depression.

Hey, even I see those numbers and shake my head. There are going to be nights when it will be tough to squeeze in even 6 hours. So remember this: Sleep quality is just as important as the total number of hours you're under the covers. Things like caffeine, alcohol, and late-night TV can keep you from feeling reenergized when the alarm goes off. So, especially on nights you may be skimping, keep an eye on those things to ensure that you're getting the best quality of sleep—no matter how many hours you manage to fit in.

One question I hear from a lot of

KEEP IT IN CHECK

A study conducted by researchers at the University of Colorado Sleep and Chronobiology Laboratory found that people who were limited to just 5 hours of sleep over the course of 5 days gained, on average, nearly 2 pounds. But there are two slightly more subtle points of the study that are worth highlighting: All the participants had access to unlimited amounts of food, and they also weren't told to try to watch their intake. You can fend off the reported weight gain by tackling both: Keep high-calorie snacks and treats out of the house, and keep your weekly and long-term goals in plain sight. (Try writing them down and sticking them on the fridge.)

women is, "Should I exercise in the morning even if I'm dead tired?" I know the feeling because I struggle with it all the time. If you truly didn't get enough shuteye (you rolled in at 3 a.m. or were up all night with a crying baby), crawl back under the covers. Research has found that when dieters were sleep deprived they lost less body fat and more lean muscle mass than when they tallied more Zs. What's more, exercising when you're too drained can take your focus off proper form, increasing your risk of injury.

If you're just feeling groggy, get your butt out of bed, but give yourself an out. Commit to doing half of your workout—or even one set of it. Knowing that you can cut it short will get you out the door, which is the hardest part. (On a few super-sleepy mornings, I have served up this compromise: I have to get to the gym, but if I'm still not feeling it when I get there, I can just shower and get ready for work.) Chances are, you'll pick up steam as you go and feel energized enough to finish. (I've never actually taken my shower-only shortcut.)

NIGHT LIGHT

If you love to read on your tablet, know this: A study in *Applied Ergonomics* found that using a tablet for 2 hours suppresses the production of melatonin—a hormone necessary for sleep—by 23 percent. Here's how to get in a chapter before bed *and* a full night of Zs.

» Limit yourself to 1 hour and turn off other lights in the room.
» Invest in a filter that blocks shortwave blue-light emissions.
» Set your tablet to display large white text on top of black.

STOP STRESSING

No, seriously, I get it: Your daily commute. Your in-laws. Your bank statement. Your never-ending to-do list. Life is hard. But when you get all bent out of shape about any of these daily stressors, it's not just your mood that takes a hit. Your body has a physical reaction, as well. That headache-inducing, anxiety-producing feeling is your body's way of trying to maintain balance in the midst of the madness, which it deals with in the only way it knows how: by signaling your adrenal glands to release the stress hormones cortisol and adrenaline (which docs call epinephrine).

You may be more familiar with adrenaline as the fight-or-flight hormone; it gives you instant energy so you can get out of (what your body perceives as) harm's way. But then there's cortisol, which is released by your adrenal glands and may interfere with the signals that control appetite (ghrelin) and satiety (leptin), research suggests. As if that's not bad enough, cortisol inhibits the muscle-repair process and alters your metabolism so that your body stores more calories as fat instead of burning them off. Case in point: Women having a stressful day burned an average of 104 fewer calories after eating one high-fat meal compared with their nonstressed peers—a difference that could result in a weight gain of almost 11 pounds per year. Even worse, that fat tends to settle around your waistline, because visceral fat—or intra-abdominal fat, which resides underneath the abdominal muscles—has more cortisol receptors than fat below the skin.

Here's the great news: You don't have to resign yourself to feeling frazzled. The key is remembering that stress is about your mindset: What distinguishes one person's meltdown from another's composure is their perception of control over the situation. When you start to feel tensions rise, take control by utilizing a proven stress-busting strategy.

TEA OFF

In a study at University College in London, volunteers drank the equivalent of a cup of black tea before completing two stressful tasks. Afterward, their cortisol levels dropped an average of 47 percent, compared with 27 percent for the people who didn't imbibe.

JUST SAY "%&* IT!"

Swearing reduces stress, according to research published in the *Leadership & Organization Development Journal.* Now, I'm not saying that gives you a pass to drop F-bombs in the middle of your office, but a strategically placed expletive in the privacy of your car, kitchen, or bedroom can help you blow off steam.

PRESS THE ISSUE

Acupressure is a quick and effective tension reliever—it can reduce stress by up to 39 percent, according to researchers at Hong Kong Polytechnic University. For fast relief, massage the fleshy area between your thumb and index finger for 20 to 30 seconds.

TREAT YOURSELF

Flavonoids in cocoa relax your body's blood vessels so that arteries can dilate, reducing blood pressure, according to a study published in the *Proceedings of the National Academy of Sciences.* Look for dark chocolate or cocoa powder, which have more of the stress-busting compounds than milk chocolate, and keep it to one serving.

TAKE A YOUTUBE TIME-OUT

Just the anticipation of laughing significantly decreases levels of the stress hormones DOPAC, cortisol, and epinephrine, according to researchers at Loma Linda University in California.

CHEW THE FAT

According to a study from the University of Pittsburgh, people with the highest blood levels of EPA and DHA omega-3 fatty acids are happier, less impulsive, and generally more agreeable. Boost your mood by adding foods rich in omega-3s—salmon, herring, and sardines top the list. Or try a daily supplement of 400 milligrams each of EPA and DHA fish oils.

DRINK UP

Water may very well be one of the most undervalued nutrients. And yet, research shows that about 41 percent of US women ages 20 to 50 don't drink enough water—roughly 74 ounces per day, or 9 cups, according to the Institute of Medicine's recommendations. Proper hydration improves exercise performance (according to researchers at the University of Connecticut, people could do 17 percent more reps in three sets when they were well hydrated), lubricates your joints, and even keeps your skin healthy and glowing. It's also critical to dropping weight—so even if you're killing it at the gym, you could be negating the calorie-burning advantages if you aren't drinking enough H_2O. Turns out, well-hydrated cells may actually boost your metabolism: After women upped their water consumption to 1 liter a day for a year, 5 pounds of their weight loss was credited to the water.

What's more, dehydration (even when it's mild) can take a toll on your mood, reports the *Journal of Nutrition*. When researchers had study participants walk on a treadmill for 40 minutes, they found that losing as little as 1 percent of body weight in fluid led to decreases in mood, concentration, memory, and energy.

And before you reach for that snack because you're "hungry," pause and drink a glass of water: If you've been eating regularly, what you perceive as hunger might actually be thirst.

MASSAGE YOUR MUSCLES

A post-workout massage isn't just an indulgence—research shows that it boosts strength recovery by 60 percent, and it may be one of the most effective strategies for preventing pain and injury.

Remember those tiny microscopic tears in the muscle fibers caused by your workouts? As they repair and try to heal themselves, patches of scar tissue can form—those "knots" in your muscles that hurt like hell. For the muscle to regain maximum strength and flexibility, the scar tissue needs to become aligned and integrated with the muscle fibers. That's where massage comes in: It reduces inflammation in the tissue and increases blood flow to the area— two things that speed up recovery and help "smooth out" any kinks.

The hands-on approach helps another part of your body that you may not know about. When your muscles are chronically tight, the surrounding fascia tightens along with them. Never heard of fascia? It's a cobweblike casing of connective tissue that surrounds every muscle, tendon, ligament, nerve, and bone in your body; it keeps each internal body part separate and allows it to slide easily with your movements. To experts like Todd Durkin, fascia quality plays a critical role in performance, joint stability, injury, and chronic pain— and it's something we don't pay nearly enough attention to.

In its healthy state, fascia is smooth and supple and slides easily, allowing you to move and stretch in every direction with a full range of motion. But it's not just like plastic wrap; fascia reacts to stress and can tighten—as it does in response to repetitive motions, trauma and injury, or even poor posture—and, over time, the fascia becomes rigid, compressing the muscles and nerves it surrounds. Sticky adhesions form between fascial surfaces, and they can be tough to eliminate. Unfortunately, our bodies don't have a natural mechanism for getting rid of them.

By correcting (aligning and smoothing out) areas of scar tissue and other muscular irregularities, massage and self-massage techniques break the muscular pain cycle at its root, accelerate healing, and restore muscular balance.

Using a foam roller on your fascia is different than using one on your muscles. Fascia works in slower cycles than muscles, both contracting and stretching more slowly. Be gentle and slow in your movements, and when you find an area of tension, hold sustained pressure for 3 to 5 minutes. Practice self-massage with the same rules. For the best results, use long, smooth strokes over your muscles. If you find a knot, move slowly from the outside in, but keep the pressure light. If any areas feel particularly tight or sticky (a sign of adhesions), spend extra time stretching and massaging there to prevent a future injury. For acute soreness, apply a cold compress or ice pack for about 20 minutes to further decrease inflammation.

GET MOVING

You may feel like rewarding yourself with some downtime, but doing a low-key activity the day after a big workout will prolong the muscle-sculpting perks of increased circulation. Fresh blood flow brings fresh nutrients to your muscles and helps flush waste products. What's more, staying active has also been proven to reduce post-exercise muscle soreness and suppress nervous-system activity that can result in poor sleep.

Take a restorative yoga class or go on a walk with friends at a conversational pace. If you're sitting behind a desk all day, stroll around the office for about 10 minutes every couple of hours to get things moving. Then prepare for a different kind of reward: a less-painful gym session tomorrow.

WORK OUT THE KINKS

In one survey, 45 percent of respondents said sore, tired muscles keep them from working out more often. Loosen up with a foam roller: A study in the *Journal of Strength & Conditioning Research* found that just 2 minutes of rolling is enough to improve recovery in quadriceps muscles. And that benefit continues throughout your entire body. Tend to aching muscles with this foam-roller routine. The moves take 10 to 15 minutes to complete and hit all your soreness-prone places. Plus, you can do them anytime: during your favorite

TV show, before bed, first thing in the morning, or after a workout. Roll over each spot 5 to 10 times. If a spot feels extra tender, try this: Start below the area, work up to it and hold for a few seconds, and then roll through it.

CALVES / Sit on the floor with your legs straight out, hands on the floor behind you supporting your weight. Place the foam roller under your calves (A). Slowly roll up and down along the backs of your legs, from your knees to your ankles (B).

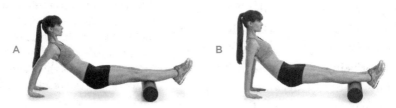

HAMSTRINGS / Sit with your right leg on the roller; bend your left knee, cross your left ankle over your right ankle, and put your hands on the floor behind you (A). Roll up and down from your knee to just under your right butt cheek (B). Switch legs.

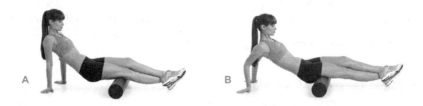

QUADS / Lie facedown on the floor, cross your calves, and place the roller under your hips (A). Lean on your right leg (B) and roll up and down from your hip to your knee. Switch legs.

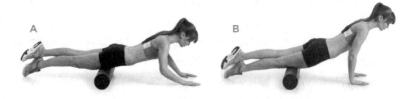

BACK / Sit on the floor with the foam roller under your lower back, resting your hands behind you for balance, legs bent and feet flat on the floor (A). Tighten your abs and slowly bend your knees to move the roller up your back, to just below your shoulder blades (B).

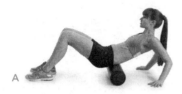 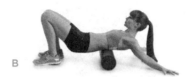

HIPS AND OUTER THIGHS / Lie on your side with the roller under your right hip, your left foot on the floor in front of you (A). Bracing your abs and glutes for balance, slowly roll down from your hip to your knee (B). Switch to the other side and repeat.

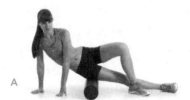 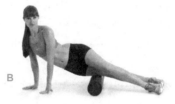

SHOULDERS AND LATS / Lie on your back with the roller behind your shoulders, legs bent and feet flat on the floor. Lace your fingers loosely behind your head and lean your upper back into the roller (A). Brace your abs and glutes for stability, and slowly press into the roller on your left side, raising your right shoulder (B). Roll from your underarms to the bottom of your rib cage. Return to the center and switch sides.

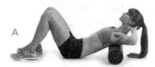 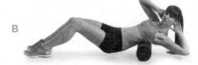

BUTT / Sitting on the roller, cross your right leg over your left knee and lean toward your right hip, putting your weight on your hands for support (A). Slowly roll your right butt cheek over the roller (B). Switch sides.

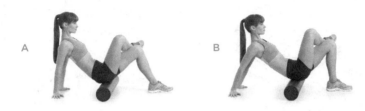

FIX YOUR POSTURE

Your mom may have told you that slouching was merely poor manners, but poor posture can actually prevent you from getting the body you're after, despite any amount of exercise. (I bet that got you to sit up straight.)

That's because over time, poor posture takes a serious toll on your spine, shoulders, hips, and knees. In fact, it can cause a cascade of structural flaws throughout your body that lead to back and joint pain, reduced flexibility, and compromised muscles—all of which limit your ability to burn fat and build strength.

Poor posture could also be to blame if you're prone to side stitches during workouts. Research in the *Journal of Science and Medicine in Sport* found that people who round their upper backs are more prone to these crippling cramps and feel more intense discomfort. The reason: A hunched posture may compress the nerves that run along your spine and into your belly, making people who hunch more sensitive to pain.

STRAIGHTEN UP

Stand taller (and look slimmer) with these simple fixes for some of the most common posture problems from Bill Hartman, PT, CSCS, co-owner of Indianapolis Fitness and Sports Training.

FORWARD HEAD / You need to address the stiff muscles in the back of your neck. Moving only your head, drop your chin down and in toward your

Sure, hunched shoulders are easy to spot, but not all postural issues are as easy to pinpoint. Wear something form-fitting and have someone snap two full-body photos of you—one from the front and one from the side. Relax your muscles and stand as tall as you can, feet hip-width apart. Then use the exercises in the next section to improve any problems you uncover.

FROM THE FRONT

1. Look at your shoulders. One shouldn't appear higher than the other.

2. Check out your kneecaps. Do they point inward, causing your knees to nearly touch when your legs are straight?

3. Do your toes point outward more than 10 degrees? This means you're duck-footed.

FROM THE SIDE

1. If your ear is in front of the mid-point of your shoulder, your head is too far forward.

2. Can you see your shoulder blades? This means your back is rounded.

3. If your lower spine is arched significantly and your hips tilt forward (you may have a belly pooch, even if you don't have an ounce of fat on your body), this means you have an anterior pelvic tilt.

sternum while stretching the back of your neck. Hold for a count of 5; do this 10 times a day.

ROUNDED SHOULDERS / Weakness in the middle and lower parts of your trapezius (the large muscle that spans your shoulders and back) is the main culprit. While it might not seem like a big deal, rounded shoulders compress your ribs and abdomen, making your torso appear wider than it actually is. To fix it, lie facedown with your arms overhead in a Y position on the floor. Squeeze your shoulder blades together and raise your arms a few inches off the floor; hold for 2 or 3 seconds, then return to the starting position. Do two sets of 12 reps.

ANTERIOR PELVIC TILT / You've got tight hip flexors. (Welcome to the club—it's an incredibly common issue, especially for women who run and bike often or who sit behind a desk all day every day.) Meet your new main move: Kneel on your left knee with your right foot on the floor in front of you, knee bent. Press forward until you feel the stretch in your left hip. Tighten your butt muscles on your left side until you feel the front of your hip stretching comfortably. Reach upward with your left arm and stretch to the right side. Hold for a count of 30 seconds. That's 1 rep; do 3 on each side.

ELEVATED SHOULDER / This happens most often when the muscle under your chest (running from your ribs to your shoulder blades) is weak. Here's a simple move you can do to remedy it: Sit upright in a chair with your hands next to your hips, palms down on the seat, arms straight. Without moving your arms, push down on the chair until your hips lift up off the seat and your torso rises. Hold for 5 seconds. That's 1 rep; do two or three sets of 12 reps daily.

PIGEON TOES / You'll see this a lot with women who have weak glutes (butt muscles). Make this a new daily staple: Lie on one side with your knees bent 90 degrees and your heels together. Keeping your hips still and heels together, raise your top knee upward, separating your knees like a clamshell. Pause for 5 seconds, then lower your knee to the starting position. That's 1 rep. Perform two or three sets of 12 reps on each side.

DUCK FEET / You might be spotting a theme here: Many foot and lower-body posture issues stem from an imbalance between the muscles in your core. Duck feet signal that your oblique muscles and hip flexors are weak. Fix it: Get into a pushup position with your feet resting on a stability ball. Without rounding your lower back, tuck your knees under your torso, using your feet to roll the ball toward your body, then back to the starting position. That's 1 rep. Do two or three sets of 6 to 12 reps daily.

IMPROVE YOUR POSTURE—ALL DAY LONG!

Proper form isn't only important during your workouts. There are endless situations throughout the day that can hurt your posture—and we hardly give them a thought. Here's the best, and safest, way to . . .

PICK UP A TODDLER / Bend your knees—so as not to strain your hips, spine, or neck—and crouch all the way down to eye level with the child. Pull the munchkin close to your body—as in a hug—and slowly stand straight up.

STAND AT A COCKTAIL PARTY / Keep your knees slightly bent and your weight over your entire foot. High heels shift your weight forward, so consciously think about having your weight in your heel. Change your stance every few minutes.

DRIVE A CAR / With your neck and shoulders relaxed, lightly grip the steering wheel at 10:00 and 2:00, à la your driving-school days. Move your eyes independently of your head—there's no need for too much neck movement.

SIT AT YOUR DESK / Center yourself on your sit bones, then think about your spine drawing straight up toward the ceiling and your shoulders extending outward. Keep your neck long and still, and get up and move every 15 minutes to stay loose.

WASH DISHES / To reach into an overflowing sink full of dishes, hinge forward from your hips (like you're sticking your butt out to close a car door behind you), rather than hunching down with your shoulders or upper back. Move your head, neck, and torso as a single unit so that your spine stays long.

QUICK TIPS:
LIGHTER BITES

116 Snack smart. People who were served a small, healthier snack with a small amount of junk food were as satisfied as those who were given a larger serving of the treat, say study authors. Try these pairs to curb the urge to overeat.

9 baby carrots and 8 cheese curls

1 fruit cup (in 100 percent juice) and 1 chocolate chip cookie

1 side salad and 8 fries

1 side of steamed vegetables and ½ cup of mac and cheese

117 Go big at breakfast. Research has found that study participants ate more cereal, by weight, when the flakes were little—216 calories when the size of the flakes were approximately 1 inch, versus 296 calories when the flakes were 60 percent smaller. Small pieces fill a bowl more densely, making it harder to gauge how much you're actually eating, study authors say.

118 Watch the add-ons. Piling even healthy toppings onto your salad can add hundreds of calories. Try to stick with one or two extras, and keep these portions in mind.

Dried cranberries: ⅓ cup = 123 calories

Feta cheese: ¼ cup = 99 calories

Sunflower seeds: ¼ cup = 102 calories

French dressing: ¼ cup = 286 calories

119 Say cheese wisely. Sub out a slice of American with an ounce of goat or feta cheese and you'll save 17 calories and 1 gram of fat.

120 Go splits. Can't give up your sugary cereal? Slowly dial back by adding a percentage of a healthier pick. So, instead of having 1 cup of the sweet stuff, combine $\frac{1}{2}$ cup of it with $\frac{1}{2}$ cup of a healthier option, such as Fiber One.

121 Eat some chocolate. According to a new study in the journal *Nutrition*, subjects who ate about $1\frac{1}{2}$ ounces of chocolate per day had lower BMIs, less body fat, and trimmer waists, on average, than those who nibbled less. The treat contains catechins—compounds that are believed to help regulate hormones related to obesity, say study authors. Catechin levels rise with the cocoa content, which means the darker you go, the better.

122 Open a window. Nothing smells as good as the scent of cinnamon and sugar wafting through your kitchen, but allowing the scent of home-baked treats to linger for hours can trigger you to eat more. Crack a window to air out the tempting aroma.

IMPATIENCE NEVER COMMANDED SUCCESS.

FITNESS FIX

15/

What
a Pain
in the . . .

SOME SORENESS IS TO be expected with exercise—especially for beginners or people kicking up their intensity—but you don't need to take the whole "no pain, no gain" mantra so literally. Women runners, for example, tend to push through pain more than men do, which leads to injuries that could have been prevented. That's not being tough—frankly, it's stupid. Nothing will stop you short of your goals quicker than being sidelined with an injury.

LISTEN TO YOUR BODY

Kicking ass at boot camp or during your treadmill sprints does no good if it lands you on the couch for the rest of the day—or week. This is when it really counts to listen to your own body—and adjust accordingly. Paying attention to how you feel, particularly your soreness and energy levels, turns out to be a pretty accurate gauge of how prepared your body is for your next workout, according to a study in the *Journal of Strength and Conditioning Research*. Keep it mind that it's not just your workout that causes your body to feel stress and fatigue: Everyday "life stuff"—whether it's deadlines at work, a poor night's sleep, or a fight with your significant other—contributes to how well your body can bounce back after exercise. So don't just go by how you *think* you should feel because of a workout. Tune in to how you *actually* feel, then use this simple scale to decide how hard you should push yourself.

If your muscles ache and you feel completely wiped out: You'd be considered a 1 or 2 (aka very poorly or not well recovered). Your best bet is to take a rest day or do a light active-recovery workout. (Go for a walk or do some yoga or foam rolling.)

If you're a little stiff and tired, but you feel generally strong: Think of yourself as a 5 or 6 (somewhat to moderately recovered). Go ahead with your regularly scheduled workout, but pay extra-close attention; if a specific move or speed causes discomfort, back off.

If you feel fresh, energized, and ready to go: Rate yourself a 9 or 10 (very well or completely recovered). This is the time to feel free to amp up your workout—push the pace 20 percent harder or go 20 percent longer during cardio.

And remember, attitude is everything: A rosy outlook could mean fewer exercise injuries: Experts found that athletes with an optimistic disposition were less likely to be sidelined with a strain, tear, or other ache over a 2-year period than those who were less optimistic. Try adopting a few habits practiced by happy people, which are most likely the key to their low injury rates: Ease into new workouts, sleep well, and eat right. If you do get injured, focus on the positive; concentrate on the goal of getting better, say study authors.

WATCH FOR POWER STRUGGLES

Nearly every major muscle group in your body has a corresponding group that carries out the opposite function. Take your biceps and triceps: Their even matchup lets you bend and straighten your elbow without any thought. At least, that's how it should work.

Unfortunately, everyday habits (like sitting at a desk), repetitive workouts (say, that marathon you're training for or your three-times-a-week spin class), and even your wardrobe (I'm looking at those skyscraper heels) threaten these partnerships. The result: One of the muscles becomes stronger and overpowers the other, a common condition known as muscular imbalance.

Like any team, if one area is weak, another part must pick up the slack, and the entire system suffers. The danger of muscular imbalances is that they alter your natural movement patterns. Over time, they can pull bones and joints out of alignment, which often leads to pain and injury.

They can also worsen poor posture and wreak havoc on your figure. (Tight hip flexors, for example, can tilt your hips forward and give the look of a stomach pooch.) Correcting imbalances helps elongate your silhouette and can make you look 5 pounds lighter.

The fix isn't as simple as isolating the pair and strengthening the weak muscle while leaving the other alone. That's because muscles, ligaments, tendons, and bones are all connected and dependent on each other through an intricate system that's known by trainers and doctors as the kinetic chain. This system relies on the cooperation of two interrelated principles to promote movement throughout your body: stability, which allows muscles, tendons, and ligaments to hold a joint in position; and mobility, which permits both the joint to safely move through a full range of motion and the nearby muscles to cause that motion. Because the collection of parts functions as a whole, when one of those elements is lacking in one area of your body, it throws off the rest of your body. That means your back pain could actually stem from a problem with your shoulder, your knee, or even your shin.

That said, knowing what imbalances you may have can help ID what's causing your pain—and spotting them early can mean preventing future injuries. Here are simple self-tests on three common female imbalances. If an area is out of whack, work the fix into your total-body routine at least three times a week.

CHEST VERSUS BACK

A balanced upper body helps you stand taller, look leaner, and stave off shoulder and back pain. Problem is, many women prioritize their arms and abs over their backs and chests. Combined with spending hours hunched over a keyboard, this imbalance can cause what experts call a protracted shoulder girdle (what you know as rounded shoulders and slouchy posture). It's a sign that the muscles on the front of your body are tight, while your back muscles are weak. To test it, lie faceup with your arms by your sides, palms facing in. Raise your arms overhead until they touch the floor. If your back arches, your palms turn toward the ceiling, your elbows point outward, or you can't touch your arms to the floor, you need to improve this imbalance.

**THE FIX / LYING
DUMBBELL PULLOVER** Lie
faceup on a bench, feet flat on the floor,
holding a pair of dumbbells directly
over your chest, arms completely
straight (A). Keeping your arms
straight, brace your core and lower the
weights toward the floor as far as you
can, or until your arms are in line with
your ears (B). Pause, then raise the
weights back to the starting position.
That's 1 rep. Do 10 to 12.

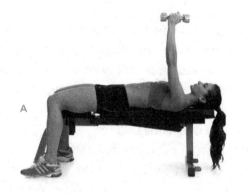

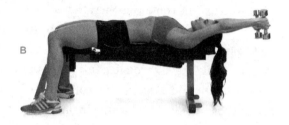

QUADRICEPS VERSUS HAMSTRINGS

Out of the biological gate, women are more likely to be quad dominant (meaning they use their quads more than their hamstrings) than men are. Wider hips throw off lower-body alignment and make it difficult for the posterior muscles, like your hamstrings, to work properly. This imbalance is made worse by thigh-centric workout programs that emphasize the quads—two of many women's go-to lower-body moves are lunges and squats.

Striking a more even balance can lower your risk for injury as well as increase your running speed and overall power. A study in the *American Journal of Sports Medicine* found that 70 percent of athletes with recurring hamstring injuries suffered from muscle imbalances between their quadriceps and hamstrings. After correcting the imbalances by strengthening the hamstrings, every person in the study went injury free for the entire year after. Test it by standing in front of a chair that's a foot away from a wall, your toes 6 inches from the wall, feet hip-width apart, and arms raised overhead.

Keeping your arms overhead and chest upright, squat into the chair. If you lose your balance, raise your heels off the floor, or touch the wall, you likely have dominant quads.

THE FIX / STABILITY BALL LEG CURL AND KNEELING QUAD STRETCH

Lie on the floor with your calves on a stability ball (A). Raise your hips, then pull the ball toward you (B). Return to the starting position. That's 1 rep. Do 10 to 12. Then kneel in front of a step or bench, placing one foot flat on the floor in front of you. Raise your back foot and place it against the step or bench (C). Hold for 15 to 20 seconds, then switch sides and repeat.

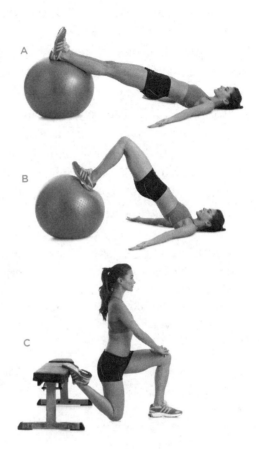

A

B

C

GLUTES VERSUS HIP FLEXORS

Your glute muscles are the powerhouse of your lower half, plus they help stabilize your hips and pelvis, keeping your spine properly aligned. Yet most people don't train them nearly as much as they should. What's more, over time, sitting around too much causes your glutes to lose strength and eventually even to forget how to contract (or, as *Women's Health* fitness expert Rachel Cosgrove says, to develop "gluteal amnesia"). At the same time, your hip flexors—the muscles that connect your hip bones to your legs—become short and stiff. This couch-potato combo tilts your pelvis forward, which increases the arch in your back and puts stress on your spine. From a cosmetic standpoint, it pushes your abdomen out, making even a relatively flat stomach bulge. Here's how to check for it: Lie on a bench, knees at your chest. Holding one knee, lower the other leg as far as possible while keeping it straight. Switch legs. If either leg doesn't rest on the bench, you likely have tight hip flexors (a sign of weak glutes).

THE FIX / GLUTE BRIDGE AND SCORPION

Lie faceup with your knees bent, feet flat on the floor (A). Raise your hips toward the ceiling (B); pause, then lower. That's 1 rep. Do 12 to 15. Then lie facedown on the floor with your legs straight (C). Raise your right foot off the ground, bending your knee, and reach your toe to the left, lifting your right hip off the ground while keeping your upper body still (D). Hold for 3 seconds, then slowly reverse the movement to return to the starting position; that's 1 rep. Repeat on the other side and continue alternating for 10 to 12 total reps.

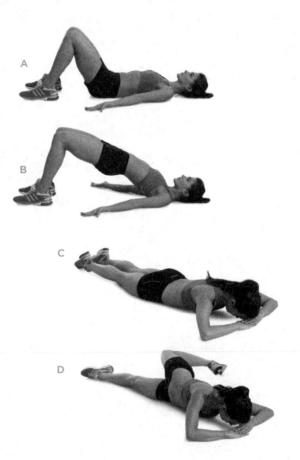

THE COST OF HIGH HEELS

Your high-heel habit comes at a price. For starters, wearing them shifts your weight forward, placing more stress on your quads and less on your hamstrings and glutes (which doesn't help the imbalance you just read about). Plus, when you elevate your heels chronically, your ankle mobility—your toe-to-shin range of motion—suffers. This might not sound like a big deal, but it can actually cause a number of problems further up the kinetic chain.

It can also lead to a muscular imbalance between your calf and shin muscles. Strong shin muscles may not get you noticed in short shorts, but this small muscle is critical for controlling your foot landing. When it's weak, your calf muscles must absorb the extra shock, which can lead to shin splints. Wearing high heels makes it worse: Women who wore 2-inch heels (or higher) for at least 40 hours a week for at least 2 years walked differently than those who usually wore flats, according to a study in the *Journal of Applied Physiology.* If your foot is forced into a position in which your toes point downward, your shin muscles get weaker, your calf muscles get shorter, and your Achilles tendon gets stiffer, which could lead to injuries over time. Use these three tips to help fix the issue.

STRETCH YOUR CALVES / Researchers found that people who sprain their ankles don't have the same range of motion in those joints as folks whose ankles stay injury-free. Tight gastrocnemius and soleus muscles limit ankle motion.

TAKE A BREAK / If you can, only wear towering heels once or twice a week, and kick them off while sitting at your desk.

ADD TOE RAISES / Using a chair for balance, slowly raise your toes off the ground; slowly lower them. That's 1 rep. Do 15 to 20.

DECODE YOUR INJURY

Luckily, the most common exercise aches and pains can be spotted and treated at home. Use this guide from Jordan Metzl to keep injuries at bay. (Red-flag exceptions: Go see a doctor if you've experienced a sudden trauma such as a fall or if the pain keeps you up at night or lasts longer than 2 weeks.)

LOWER BACK (OR UPPER BUTT)

WHAT IT COULD BE / Piriformis syndrome (a tight butt muscle) or a herniated disk (some are worse than others). Both injuries put pressure on the sciatic nerve in your back. The jury's out on what causes piriformis syndrome, but a herniated disk is often the result of improper lifting form or sports that involve rotating.

DIY TREATMENT / Take an OTC pain reliever, rest when you feel sore, then hit the gym. One study found that non-weight-bearing exercise (such as riding a stationary bike) and core training relieve back pain better than lying in bed.

SEE THE DOC IF . . . You also have a fever, leg weakness, or bladder changes. These symptoms may signal an infection or nerve compression.

ELBOW

WHAT IT COULD BE / Inflammation of the lateral epicondyle tendon (tennis elbow) or the medial epicondyle tendon (golfer's elbow). Swinging a racket or club is the obvious culprit, but any activity that involves the elbow (like softball) can tax its tendons.

DIY TREATMENT / Swallow an OTC pain reliever, ice your elbow, pick up a brace at your local pharmacy to stabilize the tendons, and ease yourself back on course (or court).

SEE THE DOC IF . . . You have trouble moving your elbow normally or rotating your palm up and down, or if you have severe swelling and bruising at the joint.

KNEE

WHAT IT COULD BE / Pain on the outside of the knee signals an inflamed or tight iliotibial band (IT band), the tissue that runs from hip to knee. Pain around the kneecap could be runner's knee—a wearing away of the cartilage under the kneecap. Increasing distance or speed too suddenly is the most common cause of an IT band injury, but research suggests it's also associated with weak hip abductors and glutes. Runner's knee is the result of overtraining, improper running form, or weak quads and hip muscles.

DIY TREATMENT / Loosen your IT band with this move: Lie on your side and support your weight with your forearm. Slip a foam roller under your hip and slowly roll down from hip to knee. Repeat this a few times a week. For runner's knee, reduce your mileage to a point that doesn't cause pain, and do leg lifts and presses to strengthen your quads and hamstrings.

SEE THE DOC IF . . . Your knee is very swollen or gives out. These signs point to a tear of the anterior cruciate ligament (ACL) or meniscus (knee cartilage).

HEEL

WHAT IT COULD BE / Plantar fasciitis—inflammation of the connective tissue at the bottom of the foot, which helps support your arch. The usual suspects include overtraining, running on hard surfaces, and wearing worn-out running shoes.

DIY TREATMENT / OTC gel heel inserts may help reduce pain and swelling, and street runners may feel relief after switching to a treadmill or trail.

SEE THE DOC IF . . . You have severe pain directly after an injury, or if you're unable to rise up on your toes or walk normally.

SHIN

WHAT IT COULD BE / Medial tibial stress syndrome (better known as shin splints). The "terrible toos" (too much, too soon, too often, too fast, too hard) are usually to blame.

DIY TREATMENT / Switch to a non-weight-bearing exercise such as swimming or biking for 2 weeks, and ice the area for 20 minutes after each session.

SEE THE DOC IF . . . Pain is localized on the outer edge of the shinbone. You may have a stress fracture.

ANKLE

WHAT IT COULD BE / A sprain, which happens when the ligaments are stretched beyond their normal range. You might have rolled your ankle while playing tennis or soccer, or you stepped in a pothole.

DIY TREATMENT / Do the RICE method: Rest; ice for 20 minutes three times a day; compress with an elastic bandage; and elevate your foot above heart level as much as possible for 48 hours.

SEE THE DOC IF . . . You can't put any weight on the injured foot, or if it's still swollen and painful after 3 days.

QUICK TIPS:
ACHES & PAINS

123 **Show your feet some TLC.** A survey by the American Podiatric Medical Association found that 77 percent of Americans have experienced foot pain, and 50 percent say that issues with their feet have kept them from exercising and walking. Try to keep your heels to 3 inches or less—54 percent of women surveyed were comfortable in shoes under that height.

124 **Tape it up.** Twenty-five percent of people worldwide suffer from chronic knee pain. Research suggests that applying Kinesio Tape—a therapeutic tape that supports muscles and joints—to the hip can bring relief.

125 **Stretch in the shower.** Short on time? You can skip your post-workout stretch, but try to squeeze in a stretch or two while you're showering off.

126 **Strengthen your shins.** If you want your shins to feel as good as your calves look, add toe raises to your weekly warmup routine. (Try three sets of 10 to 20 reps.) Strong shin muscles can help prevent shin splints.

127 **Don't tough it out.** If you're losing proper form, take a minute to catch your breath, and then get back into your workout at a slightly lower intensity.

128 **Keep time with your music.** The right tunes can make your workout feel less strenuous, according to a new study in the journal *Medicine & Science in Sports & Exercise.* Cyclists pedaling to music at the same speed as the tune's beat reported less discomfort—probably because focusing on keeping time with the song kept their minds off the pain, say study authors.

129 **Protect your ears.** While you're focusing on your music (not the ache in your legs), keep the volume at 60 percent and remove your earbuds after an hour.

SETBACKS ARE NOT THE SAME AS FAILURES.

FITNESS FIX

16/

Managing Your Motivation

FOR A LOT OF women I talk to, the impetus for launching into a new diet and fitness kick is some kind of aesthetic goal: to lose weight, to get a flat stomach, to tone their arms and shoulders. For some, it's their upcoming wedding; for others, it's the beach vacation they just booked with their significant other. Because they feel some incentive to look and feel their best, they're super motivated. Which is awesome! Right? Of course it is—*but* (you had to know there was a but coming) that early excitement can sometimes backfire.

DEALING WITH DEADLINES

Before starting any successful weight-loss program, you need an accurate and realistic frame of reference for how long it will take to burn body fat. Notice that I didn't say lose weight. Though often used interchangeably, these two things are not exclusively linked. (You can, in fact, lose weight at a pretty fast pace by shedding water weight and sometimes even precious fat-fighting lean muscle, which is not our goal here.) Your trim-down timeline depends on a variety of factors, including your age, gender, activity level, calories consumed, and current weight, which means your pace is going to be individualized. Keep in mind that while people with more weight to lose can see larger losses almost immediately, seeing fast double-digit drops like TV weight-loss contestants experience isn't realistic. (And those quick losses are a good sign you're losing weight, not body fat.) Of course, we all want the quickest fix, but that immediate

TAME YOUR ENTHUSIASM

When you amp up your activity levels too quickly, you may end up with disrupted sleep, increased susceptibility to colds, and fatigue, according to a study in the journal *Medicine & Science in Sports & Exercise.* To avoid this syndrome—called overreaching—increase your cardio time by no more than 10 percent per week. If you're already feeling the effects of doing too much, take a few days off from the gym, and when you return, build back up slowly: Spend only about one-quarter as much time exercising as you did preburnout, then add a few minutes to your workout every week.

. . . .

gratification pales in comparison to actually maintaining the weight loss for years after. A typical barometer for fat loss is losing up to 2 pounds a week.

How quickly you can hit your desired target depends on a number of individual factors, but the common denominator is avoiding the fitness and diet mistakes that can wind up slowing you down—or even sidelining you. Use the tips that match your time frame and goals to help you work out more effectively, and pace yourself for fast, but not fleeting, results.

While weight loss seems like a relatively straightforward equation—calories in have to be less than calories out—each goal has its own subtle but unique approach for delivering results. For example, cardio at a steady, moderate pace can help a woman who is 20 pounds overweight kick off her fitness program and see early results. But try that approach when you're single digits away from your goal and your results will likely flatline. Whatever your goal, use these guidelines to get where you want to go—quickly and effectively.

YOU WANT TO LOSE . . . 20+ POUNDS

Your goal weight may seem far off, but don't sweat it. The more you weigh, the more calories you burn during easier workouts like brisk walking. No need for killer workouts just yet: Small, consistent efforts will help you shed pounds early on—and seeing those quick results will motivate you to stay on track.

Your biggest challenge is keeping injuries at bay. Excess weight makes exercise naturally harder on your joints. Start with basic bodyweight exercises 2 days a week; they put less strain on your body and help you learn proper form. "Simple Workouts That Work: Bodyweight" on page 124 is built to adjust with you; once you master the fundamental moves, your joints and muscles will be prepped to tackle more-difficult exercises and increase to three sessions per week.

And while in most cases slow and steady isn't the best approach, it's the key to developing endurance, a crucial building block at this weight-loss stage. Sustained, moderate-intensity cardio slowly introduces your joints to impact, reducing your risk of getting injured. What's more, it helps teach your body to utilize fat as fuel so that over time you begin to burn more of it. Two days a week, aim to complete 30 to 45 minutes of easy- to moderate-intensity cardio. (You can walk, hike, bike, or swim—anything that keeps you going for at least 30 minutes.) Mix up your routine to train different muscles and beat boredom. And pay attention to your body: It's better to do too little than too much at this stage. If you're feeling fatigued, reduce the duration of a workout or take a day off.

YOU WANT TO LOSE . . . 10 POUNDS

Breaking this double-digit barrier can be frustrating. Your body adapts to exercise over time, which can cause your metabolism to fall into a lull. So if you were seeing steady results and then hit a point of slow or stalled progress, your body likely adapted to the stimulus. In short: Your body got fitter, and now your go-to routine won't cut it.

Repeat after me: The secret to sailing into double digits is strength training three times a week—and not with 3-pound dumbbells. Adding resistance helps you torch more calories during and after your workout while replacing body fat with lean muscle mass. In fact, researchers at Pennsylvania State University found that 22 percent of weight loss came from losing muscle when dieters didn't lift. It's important to track your progress during workouts. When you hit a plateau, increase one of these four things: frequency (so go from three workouts a week to four); intensity (if you've been using 10-pound dumbbells, go up to 15); time (increase your workout duration by 5 minutes); or type (if you've been doing the same routine or taking the same Pilates class, switch it up). And keep your effort in check: The goal is sustained intensity—not overall duration. A good indication that you're in the right zone during your workouts: You should be able to talk, but not easily.

YOU WANT TO LOSE . . . 5 POUNDS

It's a pretty cruel joke, if you ask me: The closer you get to your ideal weight, the tougher it is to reach it. Your body is always working to maintain its natural balance, so the more weight you lose, the harder your body works to hold on to it.

One way to shake your body out of its comfort zone is with plyometrics. These explosive moves are great muscle builders, get your heart rate up, and work multiple muscles at a time. That's what makes this megawatt routine the final piece of your weight-loss puzzle: It'll shed that last layer of fat to show off the sculpted, lean physique you've been building all along.

To beat plateaus and kick your fat-burning potential into overdrive, make your cardio as explosive as your strength training. High-intensity interval

7 DAYS TO SLIM

Don't expect miracles, but by taking a practical approach you can look and feel lighter in as little as 7 days—without wrecking your metabolism.

SUNDAY: ELIMINATE PROCESSED FOODS /
If you can't pronounce the ingredients, the food is off-limits. Or hit the produce aisle for foods with no label at all.

MONDAY: LAY OFF THE SAUCE /
Not only are alcoholic drinks dehydrating and high in calories, but they also make resisting nibbles difficult. (No shocker here: Studies prove women consume more calories after drinking.)

TUESDAY: GET A FIBER FIX /
It may be tempting to nix all carbs, but don't forgo fiber, a proven source of long-lasting satiety. Sprinkle flaxseed onto yogurt or add a few teaspoons of sliced almonds to your salad.

WEDNESDAY: BURN, BABY, BURN /
Eating steadily throughout the day can prevent hunger—which makes you want to ravage anything in sight. Aim for three small meals (300 to 350 calories each) and two snacks (100 to 150 calories each).

THURSDAY: BANISH BLOAT /
Broccoli, onions, and peppers cause gassiness and bloating. Stick to water-based produce like spinach and asparagus. Potassium-rich fruits like bananas and oranges also purge retained water.

FRIDAY: FLUSH IT OUT /
Cells retain water when they don't have enough of it. Down 2 to 3 liters each day. Sip slowly and the water will hit your bloodstream rather than filter out through your kidneys, so you won't have to pee every 5 seconds.

THE BIG DAY! BEFRIEND PROTEIN /
A healthy, protein-rich breakfast will fill you up and head off unnecessary snacking. Try one of the lightning-fast egg recipes on pages 228 to 229.

training involves quick, sprintlike bursts combined with periods of rest or easy recovery to help maximize your calorie burn. In other words, go as close to all-out as you can. Once a week, complete an interval using the cardio of your choice. Feeling good? Boost your weekly calorie burn with an extra day of cardio—30 to 45 minutes at moderate intensity (or 65 to 80 percent of your maximum heart rate).

THE SIGNS OF EXERCISE BURNOUT

Just like it's important to tune in to how you feel physically to avoid overtraining and injuries, it's just as crucial to pay attention to how you feel mentally. Like sleep, grief, and relationships, exercise—or more accurately, exercise burnout—has classic emotional stages. You're always in one of the four stages, but moving between them doesn't happen overnight and people typically don't pass through them at the same rate. Clue into the classic symptoms—and tips for how to stay on track—so you can sidestep a workout slump.

HONEYMOON PHASE

You're determined to look hot at your best friend's wedding, so you ramp up your workouts to 6 or 7 days a week—and you never miss a single session.

Which is great, but you know it can't last forever. You're actually better off taking a less-is-more approach here. Burnout often happens when you expect too much too soon, so balance your excitement with the big picture. Even with the smartest, most effective workout program, you still can't force your body to become stronger or slimmer any faster than it physiologically can. Don't exceed your ability to recover mentally or physically: Start with the lowest reps, sets, and weights. Gradually increase exercise volume and intensity to avoid injury, and always pencil in at least one full day off each week.

DISENCHANTMENT

This is the motivation backfire I was talking about: Your excitement fades when you don't see results right away. You stop looking forward to gym time and start slacking during—or flat-out skipping—workouts.

Who hasn't been there at least once? This is when finding support can be clutch: According to Penn State researchers, simply having a supportive friend, family member, or significant other makes you more likely to stick with your fitness regimen. Participants who started a new workout plan with a partner cheering them on logged more exercise hours than people who lacked this support. What's more, this is the stage where it can pay off to brag a little: According to a study published in the *Journal of Personality and Social Psychology*, when you share a triumph with someone else—like finishing a 5K or even surviving one killer abs class—and they respond enthusiastically, your perceived value of that event increases and you may become more invested in it. Plus, by sharing workout successes, you're cementing the (perhaps once-elusive) idea that exercising is part of your core identity, which can help you stay on that path.

STALLING

Assuming you can't kick yourself out of Stage 2, that downward spiral continues until you reach a point where boredom and apathy override your commitment and motivation. You'll use almost anything—work, family, stress, the weather—as an excuse to skip exercise. Sometimes you'll be fully aware you're doing it (but you just won't care enough to do anything about it). Other times, the indifference can be sneaking: You don't actually think you're making excuses, you claim; you're just really busy.

Your workout routine is dying for some of that fresh and exciting newness you felt when you got started. Nothing evaporates motivation faster than feeling like you're not making any noticeable improvements. Even if the scale hasn't budged yet and your jeans fit the same, in the early stages of a new workout routine you notice improvements. (Like, say, you're not as sore during week 2 as you were during week 1, or you finally feel comfortable doing a deadlift.) Hell, even just the fact that you have gone to the gym 3 days a week for 3 weeks is super exciting progress, initially. The problem is, once women work hard to master a new skill (like holding plank position for 60 seconds or running at a 10-minute-mile pace), they tend to stick with it—after all, it feels good to have things that once were hard feel easy. But it also impedes progress and breeds big-time boredom. You can score a big boost here by simply mixing it up: Try a new workout class (or even the same class, but with a new instructor), or go for a run with someone else and let them set the pace and distance. It doesn't have to be some huge overhaul, but those

GIVE YOURSELF A BREAK, ALREADY

There's a difference between constantly making excuses and having a little compassion for yourself when life, well, happens. When you have a more flexible and compassionate mindset for your efforts, you'll be more likely to get back on track faster than if you dwell on the "failures" and feel like you can't match the perfection that's expected.

There are dozens of possible reasons your fitness routine took a slide—maybe your work has been too crazy, you moved to a new city, or you were just feeling under the weather. It's never just about the physical roadblock; there are logistical and psychological challenges, as well. No matter where you are now, use these strategies to pave the way to a stronger, healthier body. But just remember: Maybe the most beneficial thing you can do for your long-term motivation is stop beating yourself up all the time. Progress, not perfection. Repeat it until you believe it.

Crazy work hours? Try to plan your workouts for when you have the fewest conflicts, which for most people is in the a.m. If you're committed to after-work sweat sessions, try this simple tweak: Get changed before you leave work. Otherwise, it can be tempting to head straight home—or catch the tail end of happy hour. Need more incentive? Remind yourself that daily exercise helps your mental sharpness, learning, and memory—and a recent study found that working out three or more times a week leads to higher pay, too.

Easing back in? After an injury, people either rush back into their former workouts, which puts them at risk for another injury—or are so afraid of getting hurt again that they put it off altogether. After your doctor clears you, scale back your routine by at least 50 percent for 2 weeks. Back off a bit if you begin nursing the area or feel an uptick in acute pain, which can ultimately throw off your form and cause new injuries. But at the same time, challenge those negative, "poor me" thoughts. Staying positive may sound like psychobabble, but it really works. And while it's normal to be nervous, it's important to trust your doctor's orders when he gives you the okay.

Crazy social calendar? Weeks of eating, drinking, and partying (and not exercising) can leave you feeling overwhelmed by the idea of having to undo the damage. There's this feeling of, "Oh, what the hell, it's too late now." But keep in mind, it's easier to drop 2 pounds than 10, which is what you could be facing if you delay your comeback. You don't have to give up all indulgences cold turkey, either. Make one healthy swap or change each day to ease back on track.

Moving? That's stressful. And in all the commotion, your running shoes can quickly get buried in the boxes for a little too long. Plan ahead to avoid the extra stress and make the transition easier: Scope out your fitness options before you pack the moving van. If you join the local gym or find some new running routes prior to your move, you'll have a workout plan ready once your stuff is unpacked. This lets you maintain your commitment to regular exercise—regardless of geography. To find running routes in your new neighborhood, go to usatf.org/routes.

little tweaks will bring back some novelty and challenge, which will get you more mentally engaged.

FRUSTRATION AND SURRENDER

And, the sad finish: Sometimes slowly, sometimes all at once, exercise slides from your list of top priorities. All you want to do is throw in the towel. (There's always next month—or year.)

While you may have been able to rely on internal motivation during other stages, at this point you need to call in some external reinforcements. Have you ever bribed yourself with an incentive (like treating yourself to a massage after a month of perfect gym attendance)? Behavioral economists say the flip side—penalties for missing workouts—may be even more effective. They're called commitment contracts, and when your drive to sweat is at an all-time low, they work by removing and reducing choices. Tapping into your pride can have a powerful effect. Register for a race that requires you to raise donations. You're far less likely to bail if you've already hit up your friends and coworkers to donate. Still not working? Put money on the line. Experts say people will work twice as hard when money is at stake, compared with relying only on will-power. Make a friendly wager among coworkers or friends: Everyone ponies up $20 and whoever logs the most workout sessions over 3 months wins the pot.

QUICK TIPS:
ADDING FLAVOR

130 **Flavor with citrus instead of salt.** When a savory dish needs a little oomph, try a squeeze of lemon instead of salt. A hit of citrus can make the whole recipe come to life.

131 **Spice up your leftovers.** Add hot sauce to your leftover pizza. It will taste great the next day, plus the chiles have antimicrobial properties that may help leftovers last longer.

132 **Go nuts.** For a satisfyingly thick but dairy-free soup, add some cashew cream. It's delicious and easy to make: Soak 1 cup of raw cashews in water for 6 to 8 hours, drain and rinse them, and blend with 3/4 cup water until smooth.

133 **Never throw away the cheese rind.** Drop it into a pot of soup—any kind!—for added flavor. Remove it with a spoon and discard before serving.

134 **Add some nuts.** Replace the breadcrumbs in pasta dishes with finely chopped nuts for extra flavor and a shot of protein. Try almonds on top of béchamel-based mac and cheese.

135 **Flavor it fast.** Light Italian salad dressing is a marvelous shortcut for adding flavor to homemade salsa. Add 1/4 cup to 3 cups of salsa.

136 **Add eggs for flavor.** For a creamy pasta sauce that doesn't require a ton of butter or cheese, toss a room-temperature beaten egg with the hot pasta and a little of the boiling pasta water and stir like crazy. (The heat should kill any bacteria.)

QUICK TIPS:
ADDING FLAVOR
(cont.)

137 **Skip the spray.** Many ingredients—including scallions, peppers, and nuts—require zero non-stick or taste-enhancing cooking aids, sparing you plenty of fat and calories. Just throw them in a dry pan over high heat for 5 to 8 minutes for scallions and peppers and as little as 1 minute for nuts. Heat them just until they begin to brown or become aromatic. Corn is an especially great candidate. Sweet, browned kernels form a perfect side dish or base for a fast salsa.

REMEMBER
WHY YOU
STARTED.

FITNESS FIX

17

Make It
Meaningful

REMEMBER LAJEAN LAWSON, THE woman I mentioned in the first chapter? Her words have never left me: "Being an active person is as much a state of being as a state of doing."

As I said in the previous chapter, the reason most women initially jump into a fitness or diet program is some kind of outward, physical goal. And that's great. It really is. I love seeing people get on board and get hooked. The problem is, it can be tough to transition out of the first phase of thinking—that fitness and diet are a means to an end—and into the second phase of thinking: That this is a way of life. This is who I am. It's not a tool that I'm going to pick up only when I need it and put down when I don't. It's like any important relationship in your life: Whether you love it every second of every day or not, it's not optional; it's integral.

If you want lasting change, if you want to finally get out of the up-and-down cycle of getting in shape just to get out of it, you'd better learn to believe in that fact.

RETHINKING RESULTS

How many times have you said to yourself during a workout, "I'm getting nowhere!" Nothing evaporates motivation faster than feeling like you're not making any noticeable improvement or changes. The problem is, true change—significant change—takes time.

If you get too caught up in looking down the road, you're going to find yourself frustrated and your motivation flatlining. You have to practice giving yourself props for progress.

One of the big lessons I've learned is that chasing any huge, daunting goal is a continual practice of staying in the moment. One of the most important skills to master is mental and emotional regulation during stressful situations. Why? Anxiety and panic can trigger an actual physiological response in your body that makes it more difficult to perform. When your heart starts racing during a run, zero in on what you need to do at that moment—and nothing else. Or if you start to feel overwhelmed about the process and the goal that's still months away, bring it back to the present: What do I need to do to complete today's workout to the best of my ability? By keeping the blinders on, so to speak, you can utilize your energy to keep chipping away at your goal.

While goals are good—they're what get people through everything from grueling strength workouts to marathons—sometimes the key to seeing results is shifting your focus. Especially when it comes to weight-specific goals ("I want to lose 10 pounds"), focusing only on the outcome often leads to a pattern of yo-yo exercising. Here's why: Either you get frustrated because you haven't met your goal, and you quit, or you meet your goal, quit, and gain the weight back. Keeping a magic number in mind may work temporarily, but if you want to shed extra pounds and keep them off, you need a broader goal.

Researchers have found that consistent exercisers who see working out as part of their lifestyle, rather than as a way to change their appearance, have the most success keeping weight off. So shift your focus from the scale and think of all the other ways you benefit from exercise. For example, it increases your energy, lifts your mood, and makes you feel stronger and healthier. Losing sight of your ultimate goal may actually be the real secret to staying motivated. Researchers recently reported that women who tracked immediate results after a workout—like feeling happier, more energetic, and less anxious—exercised 34 percent more over the course of a year than those who focused on weight-loss or appearance goals. It makes sense: Physical changes can take weeks and months, which can make working out feel like just another chore.

And that's important, because when it comes to managing a hectic schedule, daily to-dos that don't have tangible and immediate payoffs—including exercise—usually fall off your checklist. For an activity to feel like it's worth your time, it has to offer something very important to your daily life; otherwise it quickly begins to feel taxing and harder to justify making time for.

So give your cousin's wedding or that smaller dress size a rest for a minute and focus on these five immediate payoffs—they'll help reboot your motivation to break a sweat. Better yet: Pay careful attention to how you feel after your workouts. Are you more self-confident? Are you less stressed? Finding the payoffs that are most important to you will ensure that you prioritize exercise in your daily routine.

GET AHEAD AT WORK

Vying for a promotion? Don't sacrifice gym time for late nights at work. Researchers found that women who exercise at least twice a week feel more in control of their jobs and find them less demanding than those who don't work out. According to a survey in the *International Journal of Workplace Health Management,* workers who exercised reported a 32 percent increase in motivation and a 28 percent increase in time management compared to the days they didn't work out.

THINK SHARPER

According to a study published in *Clinical Neurophysiology,* 20 minutes of moderate exercise immediately increases attention and cognitive ability. There's a shift in brain activity that enhances executive functioning, which plans, schedules, and coordinates thoughts and actions, explain study authors. This amplified focus can last up to an hour, so schedule a quick workout during a time of day when you tend to be most distracted or before a time when you'll really need to be on point.

GET GLOWING SKIN

A pricey facial is one way to score a better complexion; a single sweat session is another. As your heart rate rises, the increase in blood flow circulates to the surface of your skin, giving you that revitalizing flush of color. Turns out, sweating is good for your skin, too: Some of the water evaporates to cool your body, and the rest is reabsorbed into your skin, giving it a nicely hydrated look post-workout.

STEP OFF THE SCALE

It can be tempting to weigh in every day, but you shouldn't. For starters, the scale can't take into account that you dropped body fat but added metabolism-boosting lean muscle mass. It's also easily swayed by daily (if not hourly) fluctuations in your water and food intake. In short, frequent weigh-ins don't always paint an accurate picture of how you're doing. If you can't stay off the scale, use it once a week. Researchers found that overweight people who weigh themselves about once a week are six times more likely to lose weight. It helps to do it on the same day and generally at the same time every week. I recommend Monday morning: Knowing you're going to be measuring your progress at the start of the week can help many women make better decisions (or at least be more conscious about the ones they're making) throughout the weekend.

HAVE HOTTER SEX

A study published in the *Journal of Sexual Medicine* found that women who completed a 20-minute treadmill run before watching an erotic film clocked a 150 percent increase in arousal. To take advantage of this, you might want to exercise at home—study authors say the swell in arousal only lasts up to 30 minutes.

SLEEP BETTER

Working out zaps stress and anxiety and helps your body regulate its own temperature—a trifecta for helping you catch more restful shut-eye. According to a study published in the journal *Mental Health and Physical Activity,* participants who engaged in moderately intense exercise for a total of 150 minutes a week (that's 30 minutes a day, 5 days a week) were able to fall asleep faster and felt less tired during daylight hours. Study authors noted that it doesn't matter what time of day you choose to fit in a sweat session, either: Only limited research suggests that late-night physical activity hurts the quality of your sleep.

SET AN INTENTION

Focusing on those "instant results" becomes even more important when we're talking about the long term. When you reach a maintenance phase (aka, you're not trying to lose weight or necessarily change anything about your figure), you at times won't feel that same fire to stay glued to your schedule as when you have a weight-loss or race deadline looming over you. I see a lot of women feeling like they always have to have an ambitious fitness goal because, after all, that goal is what kept them motivated the first time; it's the thing that kept them on track. And I get it. Without a specific goal, I've had plenty of mornings where I just do not want to get up and work out. I'll hit the snooze button a few times. I'll start rationalizing all the reasons it's totally acceptable for me to sleep in: *You don't have anything you* have *to train for right now. You had a hard spin class yesterday. You can always go after work. You can get after it even harder tomorrow.* Some of those mornings, I stay in bed. I take it as a sign that my body or mind needs some kind of break, and I don't beat myself up about it. (Because sure enough, every time I take a few days off, I find myself antsy—and yes, actually excited—to bang out a great workout.)

Other days, I push myself to just get up. *Your shoes and bag are at the foot of your bed—all you have to do is get up and go. Just go to the gym, and if you still don't feel like working out when you get there you can just shower and go to work.* I'm not always happy about it. I don't suddenly "get in the mood." But I'll just get there and do something. (I tell people all the time, use the 10-minute rule: When you really, truly don't feel like working out, commit to just 10 minutes. If you still feel like stopping after 10, fine. The mind game you're playing with yourself will usually work; you almost never actually feel like stopping, you just needed something to push you over the hump.) A lot of time that mental drag comes from two things: Not having a set plan, and not having a specific goal.

That same drag can also hit you during your workout—if you're just working out for the sake of getting exercise, or just to burn calories, or because you know you should. But consider for a moment what yoga instructors do at the beginning of class: They urge students to set an intention. Something they want to get out of the workout—like "feel more gratitude" or "let go of stress." Something that will help them stay focused and tap into the purpose of their practice. Well, experts say intention-setting can be a powerful tool in any fitness discipline, not just yoga. It zeros in on something you can connect to emotionally, and unlike a long-term goal, you can make good on an intention in a single session, which is very satisfying. And, unlike zoning out to watch the TVs above your treadmill or spacing out in between sets in the weight room, staying focused during a workout will improve your performance, boost your intensity, and amp your results. Here are a few tools that I've found are really helpful in building and maintaining a more intentional workout practice.

SILENCE YOUR INNER CRITIC

Negative mental chatter can distract you from your workout's purpose: It's tough to reduce stress while thinking that you have the biggest thighs of everyone in your cycling class. You may not even be aware of it, but defeatist or negative self-talk can damage your workout and prevent you from achieving your intention.

Don't try to clear your head or avoid thinking; just watch your thoughts. Once they actually tune in to it, many women are stunned by how often they put themselves down with negative self-talk. Over time, those critical thoughts may erode your motivation from the inside out. Keeping your head in the game helps give you the edge you need to continue working toward your intention—and your long-term goals. When I notice my mind heading into "the dark place" as I call it, I have a simple mantra: "Change the conversation."

GIVE YOURSELF A PEP TALK

Speaking of mantras: Repeating a simple word or phrase that reflects the purpose of your workout can be one of the quickest and easiest ways to stay focused on your goal. Besides being inspiring, experts say a mantra mentally hardwires your brain to enjoy exercise by acting as a cue to connect a behavior (exercise) with a reward (the positive experience of achieving your intention).

You can think of a mantra like a hashtag: #strongbodystrongmind, #yougotthis, #justkeepswimming. If you're aiming to reduce stress and anxiety, try #justbreathe as your mantra. Want to feel strong? Go with #mindovermuscle. Mentally repeat your mantra throughout your workout—especially during the really tough parts or when you catch your mind wandering.

SYNC UP YOUR WORKOUT

Plugging in your iPod during a workout might seem like an odd way to increase your focus—after all, plenty of us use music to mentally check out—but research shows that listening to certain types of tunes can actually help you keep your mind squarely on what you're doing.

Create a playlist of songs that use words or contain themes that speak to the intention that you've picked for that day's workout—and crank up the vol-

HERE'S TO THE SMALL WINS

All too often, we gloss over our smaller achievements because we don't see their value—or maybe because we worry that others won't. Instead of being excited by the 5 pounds we've lost, we fixate on the 15 we still need to drop. When talking to someone we perceive as more fit, we share our progress with qualifiers rather than confidence ("I know it's *only* a 10K . . . "). We don't even bother telling anyone about that 10-minute workout we attempted in our living room, because how embarrassing, right? It doesn't even count. This habit doesn't just undermine our progress, it undercuts our potential.

Comparison—whether it's looking too far ahead or looking around at others—can intimidate and belittle, and it can make you question why you decided to try in the first place; it can bring you to a standstill. I think continuous progress requires a bit of tunnel vision. Whatever your goal—losing weight, training for your first half-marathon, or just trying to keep up a healthy lifestyle for the next 50 years—there are countless steps between where you start and the literal or proverbial finish line. Acknowledging and celebrating the little victories along the way not only builds confidence, it also creates momentum. And you know, a funny thing happens when you turn your attention away from how far you have to go: You always feel like you get there a lot faster. And you value the journey a whole lot more.

ume when you feel like you're starting to flag. A study in the journal the *Sport Psychologist* found that tennis players recorded faster reaction times on the court when they listened to songs with an emotionally charged message (such as "Eye of the Tiger" from *Rocky III*), as compared to music with a booty-shaking rhythm but not much in the way of motivation (say, Beyoncé's "Single Ladies"). The study authors say songs with strong lyrical affirmations can give you a significant physical and mental boost when the going gets tough.

WRITE IT ALL DOWN

Making a habit of journaling each workout session can pay dividends in the long term by keeping you motivated. Research has found that the more often people log their weight and exercise, the more weight they lose (and the less they regain). Why does this work? Well, keeping a log allows you to see how far you've come and keeps you motivated to continue pushing—sort of like your own personal pat on the back. In researcher speak, this is called establishing competence, and it's at the core of the second step in fueling motivation that lasts.

There are free sites and apps like trainingpeaks.com that let you schedule, track, and analyze your workouts. (You can also find a coach or a training plan at an additional cost.) But it doesn't even have to be something that fancy. I keep a note in my phone called "2017 Training." Every time I head to the gym or finish a run or ride, I pull that up and jot down the specifics: the date, the time, where I was, and what my workout was. But here's what I think is key: I also make sure to spend a few minutes jotting down any extra notes about how I felt during the workout—mentally and physically. If my right calf was a little tight or I felt dehydrated, I write it down. Was I distracted? Was there a song that played that really got me in the mood? Did I find myself thinking about anything? Did I have an intention going in? Did I see an unexpected immediate result after? Keeping tabs on those things is what I find so incredibly meaningful. Because when you look back on a log and see a bunch of numbers, sure, that is motivating in the sense that wow, okay, look at all of the things I did. But the things I get so motivated by are notes like, "I really didn't want to do this workout today. I was tired, I'm stressed from work, I just wanted to go home. But I'm so proud of myself for showing up. And I feel amazing now that it's done."

QUICK TIPS:
MOTIVATION

138 **Think back to a top-notch workout.** According to research from the University of New Hampshire, people who tapped into a feel-good fitness moment logged more gym time than those who did not.

139 **Place your bets.** In the weight-loss race, cash may be the perfect carrot. When participants in a Mayo Clinic study were offered a chance to win—or lose—$20 a month, 62 percent completed the program, dropping an average of 9 pounds. Without monetary motivation, only 26 percent followed through, losing just 2 pounds on average. Visit sites such as HealthyWage.com and DietBet.com to set up a challenge for yourself or to make a wager with friends.

140 **Get a cheering section.** According to researchers, receiving verbal praise during your workout can actually help you perform exercises even better next time. It seems to activate the same reward circuits in the brain as major incentives (like cash) and help solidify your muscle memory for that particular skill.

141 **Pull on that spandex.** Invest in some form-fitting workout clothes. According to researchers at Springfield College in Massachusetts, most new exercisers typically go for baggy clothes. But the excess fabric hampers movement, which can make them feel even worse about themselves.

142 **Make a schedule.** Write out a manageable schedule you can stick to for at least 5 weeks. A study in *Health Psychology* reports that it takes new exercisers that long to make their sessions a habit. To prevent burnout, aim for consistent (4 or 5 days a week), moderate workouts. Too many days off in between workouts can decrease drive, especially when your deadline feels so far away. Cap each session at 30 minutes to make sure your muscles can recover.

QUICK TIPS:
MOTIVATION *(cont.)*

143 **Push through the first half.** People who pushed themselves during the first half of a workout and eased up during the second half burned 23 percent more fat than those who did the opposite, according to a study from the College of New Jersey in Ewing. The study also found that a period of moderate-intensity exercise prior to a milder one can elicit greater fat oxidation while making the overall workout feel less stressful. One more reason to get the hard part out of the way.

144 **Think of the amazing sex you will have.** Exercise can boost your sex life more than sharing a bottle of wine. Research shows that frequent exercisers have more feelings of sexual desirability.

145 **Invest in your gym wardrobe.** Yes, your gym look matters. Ditching your sloppy sweats for a more stylish outfit can increase your resolve, your mood, and even your performance.

146 **Become a morning person.** Not an early riser? Inch your alarm back a little every few days; it will gradually reset your body's clock, so you'll have more energy.

147 **Catch the weight-loss bug.** You don't have to join a weight-loss program, just be around people who do. On average, people lost 2.8 pounds in 6 months when their workplace hosted a weight-loss program—which they weren't a part of!

IMPOSSIBLE IS AN OPINION, NOT A FACT.

18/

Never Be Afraid to Go for It

BACK IN 2013, IF you had asked me if I could do an Ironman, I would have laughed at you. Don't get me wrong, I loved watching the Ironman World Championship coverage each year—seeing these athletes struggle, persist, and wring every last ounce of faith and energy out of their bodies. And for a brief moment I might have wondered what it would feel like to stand in their worn-in sneakers. But my mind always quickly snapped back to reality: I could never do that. I mean, just reading the breakdown—2.4-mile swim, 112-mile bike ride, 26.2-mile run—is exhausting. Actually doing one? Me? No, that's impossible. It was the same way I felt cheering on friends in the New York City Marathon my first year living in the city. I was moved and beyond inspired—but not in an, "Oh, I should try doing that, too," sort of way.

Then life threw me a pretty huge, completely unexpected curveball: Team Chocolate Milk asked me if I wanted to train for that same race—the 2014 Ironman World Championship in Kailua-Kona, Hawaii. With Olympic short-track speed skating legend Apolo Ohno, no less. My knee-jerk reaction was, "You've got the wrong girl." I rattled off countless reasons why: my demanding job, last year's knee surgery, my fear of swimming in open water, and, oh yeah, the fact that I hadn't once "clipped in" to a road bike or run longer than 13.1 miles.

But here's the thing: As much as I thought I should say no, I also couldn't stop thinking about it. I dissected the pros and cons with my family and friends, consulted my sports medicine doctor, and spent countless nights playing out every possible outcome in my mind. I finally realized that I needed to do what Facebook COO Sheryl Sandberg asked of all women in 2010, in her TED-Talk-turned-book-turned-social-movement: I needed to lean in. In the pages of her *New York Times* best seller, Sandberg notes: "We hold ourselves back in ways both big and small, by lacking self-confidence, by not raising our hands, and by pulling back when we should be leaning in. We lower our own expectations of what we can achieve." I could dress up my excuses with "logical" and "legitimate" explanations, but the truth was pretty plain: The only thing really holding me back was a voice in the back of my head saying, "But what if you fail?"

See, as *Women's Health* fitness director, I value (and yes, even enjoy) exercise. But in the year following my knee surgery—the first major surgery I had ever gone through—I began to doubt that I would ever get back to my previous fitness level, much less surpass it. *This is your new normal,* I thought. I didn't recognize it as being negative; I simply thought I was being realistic. Cue Sandberg's belief that women underestimate their own potential. While athletic ability is often measured by how well your muscles, heart, and lungs function, what's above the neck (aka your brain) may play a bigger role in both propelling and limiting performance. Experts agree that fear and doubt can either make us assume we aren't capable of doing something or trick us into thinking we don't really want it. Why? Simple: It can feel very vulnerable putting everything you have on the line and finding out it's still not enough—so we hold back. We unconsciously set an easier goal to protect our egos.

I never woke up with some impenetrable confidence. I was still scared as hell, but I knew I had to say yes. To call it a reaching goal would be a massive understatement. It was, without a doubt, the biggest risk I've ever taken. What followed were 6 of the most challenging, transformative months of my life. I recognized and celebrated the number of little battles I won along the way: my first race post–knee surgery; my first half Ironman; the fact that I tallied 160 days (over 271 hours!) of training—and only missed seven workouts. The lessons I learned, well, they could probably fill an entire book. But suffice it to say it was by far the greatest decision I've ever made.

I know the majority of this book has focused on how to squeeze in shorter workouts; set smaller, more manageable goals; and maintain consistency through everyday lifestyle choices. But I want to be clear: It's not because I'm against working hard or reaching past your potential. Quite the opposite. I see this book of "fixes" as the bedrock that will allow you to keep building and growing for the rest of your life. Because I think when you establish a stress-free lifestyle centered around healthy eating and exercise—when it starts to feel easy, instinctive—it frees you up to reimagine your goals. When you're not fixating on counting calories or worrying about every workout, you can put that mental and physical energy into trying something totally new—maybe even something totally intimidating. In short, you can dream bigger and do more.

When being active becomes your lifestyle, rather than a means to an end, you'll often have times where you find yourself in a pretty familiar routine—maybe it's running, or yoga, or your neighborhood boot camp. It feels challenging, but at the same time it's comfortable. It's safe. And there's nothing wrong with that. After all, that's the goal of this entire book: to help you build a consistent, unbreakable habit of healthy eating and exercise.

But just like there will be times when your motivation drops—your life priorities shift and your workouts don't find themselves at the top of the list—there may also be times when you may find yourself itching for more. Wondering, *Could I do that? Should I try that?* I'm here to tell you that you can, and you should. Without a doubt. Whatever it is. And when you find yourself in those spots, I'm here to tell you this: Never be afraid to go for it. Because I promise you, by challenging your doubts, facing your fitness fears, and reaching further—or what I like to call "leaning in to fitness"—you'll earn far more than a stronger body.

What I realized during those months training for the Ironman was that when you spend time far outside your comfort zone, fitness becomes so much more than just exercise. Sure, months of training definitely made a physical impact on me—my arms and back were more defined; my abs were as flat as they've ever been—and I won't pretend that's not a perk. But it pales in comparison to how the experience affected my outlook. I remember this one Saturday, only a few months into training, when I was 35 miles into an emotionally draining ride on my brand-new bike—and I crashed. Alone on the side of an empty road, I cried, screamed, and seriously contemplated giving up. Frustrated and defeated, I shakily rode the final 10 miles home. The next day, I fought back tears and more doubt during an overly taxing 12-mile run. I felt so embarrassed when I had to report my "failures" to my coach. I'll never forget the text he sent me in reply: "You had an epic weekend of training. Ironman is all about facing a tough challenge, and that's exactly what you did! You dug deep, and you learned a little more about what you're made of. That's why we do this."

He could not have been more right. For me, this wasn't about racing a clock or even other athletes. It certainly wasn't about trying to lose weight or shape up. It was about regaining that unshakable belief that with ordinary talent and extraordinary perseverance, no goal is out of reach.

Daring to "go big" in fitness doesn't have to mean doing an Ironman, of course. It means setting a goal that spikes equal amounts of fear and excitement in you. To go one step past what you think is possible—for yourself. And then, when you throw yourself into intimidating waters (in my case quite literally, but really with any big fitness goal), acting with confidence and deservedness—even if you have to "fake it till you make it" for a while. Because in order to achieve any goal—whether that's entering a power-lifting competition or doing a 3-day solo hike—you have to believe that you are just as capable and just as deserving as any other person. That optimistic conviction should be enough to turbocharge your performance, which in turn can boost self-expectancy. And onward and upward you go.

Years later, I can still vividly remember how it felt crossing that iconic finish line in Hawaii. I was hit with an indescribable surge of pride. I couldn't turn off the tears—or the laughter. Tears rolled down my face. *I just did that*, I thought. *I can't believe I just did that*. For months, I had been so worried about failing that I had never considered the alternative: I might succeed beyond my wildest dreams.

Going out on a limb builds confidence you didn't have before. You have to be proud of what you've accomplished, of all your hard work, of having the courage to take on a new challenge at all. And when it's all said and done, that thrill of accomplishing something you didn't think you could do inspires a confidence and satisfaction that spills over into every aspect of our lives. And that's why, again, I'll leave you with this: Never be afraid to go for it.

THE MIRACLE ISN'T THAT I FINISHED— IT'S THAT I HAD THE COURAGE TO START.

FITNESS FIX

Acknowledgments

THIS BOOK WOULD NOT have been possible without the help of so many. I'd like to take this opportunity to thank a few of them.

First and foremost, my friends and family: You guys are proof that one of the greatest gifts you can give someone is your confidence in them. Each and every time I set my eye on a big, crazy dream, you stand unwavering by my side and help me turn it into a reality. You believe in me even when I don't believe in myself and surround me (even with miles between us) with constant love and support—and that alone has made all the difference.

Mom: You taught a young Ohio girl to pride herself on being smart, strong, and driven—and gave her the confidence to chase her wildest dreams (like working for a major women's magazine in New York City). I'm a more ambitious, generous, and grateful person through your example.

Dad: Coach Steve, you have put in endless miles to make my dreams come true. You are the rock that makes me stronger, calmer, and braver; because of you, I have dared to fail, fought to find the silver linings, and pushed to never, ever give up. I promise to keep picking my head up, walking it off, and digging deep for one more "Sprint!"—no matter what life throws my way.

To the passionate fitness experts who have graciously shared their unparalleled knowledge with me all these years: Thank you for continuing to change and elevate the industry; especially to Rachel Cosgrove, Robert dos Remedios, BJ Gaddour, Mark Verstegen, Todd Durkin, Craig Ballantyne, Tony Gentilcore, Hannah Davis, Dan Trink, Mike Boyle, Bill Hartman, Valerie Waters, Andrew Kastor, Jordan Metzl, and Mike Robertson: I'm humbled by your enthusiastic support and honored by your contributions—within these pages and over the years in *Women's Health*.

To Maria Rodale, and the entire Rodale family, as well as to Gail Gonzales, Mark Weinstein, Amy King, and the rest of the books team for this incredible opportunity and for their tremendous efforts that made it a reality; to my book editor Allison Janice, for her patience, optimism, and commitment from start to finish; and to Christian O'Toole, Cathie Yun, Gabrielle Porcaro, Marissa Gainsburg, and Lauren Doyle, for all of the invaluable behind-the-scenes work that you didn't have to do, but did anyway. I'm beyond grateful and forever appreciative.

To Adam Campbell: You have been a mentor, friend, and an invaluable bank of knowledge. Without your time, attention, and patience over the years, I wouldn't be where I am today—"thank you" will never feel like enough.

To the entire *Women's Health* staff, past and present: I have been truly privileged to work beside such intelligent, supportive, and talented women. This has been my dream job, in no small part due to all of you.

And finally, to the *Women's Health* reader: All the long days and sleepless nights, all the stressful deadlines and endless edits—sometimes I wonder if it matters, if any of it actually makes a difference. Then I hear stories from you— your successes and your setbacks, your changes in mindset and your boosts in self-confidence—and it makes every ounce of effort worth it. Thank you for continuing to push me to be the very best I can be and in return, hopefully help you live out your very best life.

Index

Boldface page references denote photographs. Underscored page references denote boxed text.

Heart health
  decrease with sitting, 13–14
  increase with
    cardio, 26
    exercise, 17
    strength training, 26
  sleep amount and, 256
Heels
  on floor while lifting, _75_
  injury, 281
Herbs, storing fresh, _222_
High heels, 267, _279_, _282_
High-intensity interval training, 16, 68, 287–88
Hills, running, 192, _196_
Hip adductor/abductor machine, 65–66
Hip extensions, _74_
Hip flexors, glute imbalance with, 278, **278**
Hips
  foam rolling, 263, **263**
  strengthening, _197_
Hip thrust, 101, **101**
Holiday treats, _41_
Hot peppers, _207_
Hot potato squat, 103, **103**
Hot sauce, _293_
Hydration, 259–60

I

Iliotibial band, 66, 280–81
Immediate payoffs, from exercise, 299–300
Inactivity physiology, 13
Inchworm, 128, **128**
  with pushup, 132, **132**
Indulgences, _291_
Injury
  ankle, 281
  decrease risk
    in optimistic people, 274
    in runner's with strength training, 28
  easing back into exercise after, _291_
  elbow, 280
  heel, 281
  increase risk with
    exercise machines, 63–64, 66
    poor form, _71_
  knee, 280–81
  lower back, 280
  shin, 281
Intensity, _108_
  calorie burn and, 24
  sustained, 287
Intention, setting an, 300–304

Intervals
  high-intensity interval training, 16, 68, 287–88
  running, 192
  Tabata method, _72_
Inverted shoulder press, 85, **85**
Isolation exercises, 61
Isometric contraction, 69–70
Isometric wall squat, 125, **125**
  alternating single-leg, 129, **129**
  single-leg, 133, **133**
Italian salad dressing, _293_

J

Journaling, 303–4
Jump rope, 29, 181
Jump squat, 182, **182**, _185_
Junk food, _9_, 46, _268_

K

Kettlebell half get-up, 147, **147**
Kettlebell halo, 147, **147**
Kettlebell pushup-position row, 146, **146**
Kettlebell reverse lunge, 146, **146**
Kettlebells, 29
Kettlebell sumo deadlift, 145, **145**
Kettlebell swing, 115, **115**
  single-arm farmer's walk shuttle with, 148, **148**
Kettlebell workout, 145–48
Kinesio tape, _282_
Kinetic chain, 275, _279_
Kitchen, getting comfy in the, 29–31
Knee injury, 280–81
Kneeling quad stretch, 277, **277**
Knee pain, _74_, 280–81, _282_
Knots, 260–61

L

Lactobacillus, 214
Lateral band walk, 66, **66**
Lats, foam rolling, 263, **263**
Laughter, 259
Leafy greens, 217
Leaning in, 309–11
Leftover, _223_, _249_
Leg circles, _197_
Leg extension, banded lying, 171, **171**
Legumes, top picks for, 215–17
Leptin, 4, 258
Life expectancy, 15, 27
Light, morning, _20_
Listening to your body, 273–74